KUNDALINI RISING

Mastering Creative Energies

by
Barbara Condron
D.M., D.D., B.J.

School of Metaphysics Publishing
Timeless Wisdom, Timely Books™
Windyville, Missouri 65783

© Fifth Printing January, 2005
    First printing August, 1992. Second printing August, 1994.
    Third printing March, 1997. Fourth Printing May, 2001
by the School of Metaphysics [100147] US Copyright TX 3-575-767

Library of Congress Control Number: 93223097
Kundalini Rising : mastering creative energies / by Barbara Condron.
    Windyville, Mo. : SOM Pub., c1992. 214 p. : ill. ; 22 cm.

ISBN: 0-944386-13-X

Cover Art by David Varing and Sharka Glet
Illustrations by Dave Lappin

PRINTED IN THE UNITED STATES OF AMERICA

If you desire to learn more about the research and
teachings in this book, write to School of Metaphysics
World Headquarters, Windyville, Missouri 65783.
Or call us at 417-345-8411.
Visit us on the Internet at www.som.org
or www.dreamschool.org

Any portion of **KUNDALINI RISING: Mastering Creative Energies** may be reprinted or
reproduced in any form with the prior written permission of the Board of Governors of the
School of Metaphysics.

Contents

Introduction

Kundalini. Her name aptly conveys the mysticism that has eluded most of Mankind for centuries. Yet, she is described as a sleeping serpent coiled three and a half times at the base of your spine. In fact, her name comes from the Sanskrit *kundala* which means coiled. A storehouse of creative energy awaiting the command to spring into action, Kundalini is the active property, unconscious in most, which functions under the direction of Universal Law, DNA, and the subconscious mind. In Eastern legends she is a Goddess, and to know her is to possess the wisdom of a creator.

At a seminar on Kundalini, C. G. Jung told his colleagues the awakening of this force had rarely, if ever, been witnessed in the West. Yet, he believed the knowledge and use of Kundalini was paramount to understanding the nature of man. He suggested it would take 1000 years for Kundalini to be set into motion, and only then through indepth analysis. Jung gave this speech in 1932.

Since that time, mankind has caused his knowledge to expand rapidly through science, technology, and most importantly through communication. The world has become a neighborhood, reorganizing the consciousness of man to expand to meet the demands of newfound awareness of who we are and how we live as humanity. With each new creation, whether scientific or artistic, man is constantly changing the way he sees himself and his relationship to his creations.

Rapidly, man is realizing the need to understand the nature of his creativity to empower and insure the perpetuation of physical evolution. He is realizing the need to reach further than he ever has before, expanding creativity beyond the realm of physical manifestation alone and into the realms of spiritual consciousness. He has seen the benefits of understanding the finite world around him, building the desire to know what causes his sensory world to exist and believing himself capable of understanding these causes. Seized by a restlessness of Spirit, he is no longer content to remain unconscious of these causal forces. He is ready to explore the nature of his own creativity with full awareness and responsibility. When willing, Mankind is capable of wielding the commands to awaken the Kundalini.

Developing conscious control of Kundalini opens the thinking to higher states of creativity and deeper levels of consciousness. When uncoiled, streams of creative energy known as prana are released, drawing energy from the inner levels of consciousness for mental creation or for physical procreation. This outpouring of energy would drain the mind unless there was a means to return the used energy back into the inner levels of consciousness from whence it came. Thus the activation and use of Kundalini shares an independently intimate relationship with the mind's centers of recycling often referred to as *chakras*. After the Kundalini rises the action of the chakras must be set into motion so energy can be replenished for future creative endeavors. Exploration of the nature of the chakras brings the knowledgeable practice necessary for continued fulfillment of desires. Pursuit of the raising of the Kundalini eventually unveils the state of desirelessness which is the spiritual destiny of man.

Using creative energy as a means to manifest physical desires prepares the waking consciousness for inner revelation.

Once the awareness is awakened, the needs of the soul become paramount to our existence. When soul progression is assured through thought and action, we are ready to embrace the true meaning of Kundalini Rising. This is the involution of consciousness toward the highest ideals of mankind. One must be willing to prepare the inner Self for the full realization of Kundalini powers for she shows no grace nor mercy to the one who beckons her into action. She is merely a means to an end, a tool for man to wield in his journey toward the Spiritual enlightenment existing beyond physical creation. She is a means to elevate awareness and transcend perceived limits of our existence. With her, as it is well described in one of the world's greatest anthologies of spiritual literature, our "eyes are opened and we become as gods" living forever.

Creative Genius

Everyday, we can see the results of man's creativity in ourselves and the world around us. The book you hold in your hands is an example of singular creative endeavors unified and ordered to produce a greater creative manifestation. The author draws on her experience and understanding not only of the subject matter but of language to fill blank pages with communicated thought. The editors use what they have learned in life to streamline what is communicated and verify its contents. The artists conceptualize in picture form the ideas conveyed. The designers give this book its look and the printers reproduce it. The distributors make it available for others. The act of reading communicates the thoughts of the author to you so your experiences may be enriched. Moving this book from the mind of its creator to you is a process of many creative minds working in harmony.

The room you are sitting in is a creative manifestation of many minds. From the creators and designers of furniture to the inventor of the lightbulb, the room you occupy exemplifies an ordered and unified manifestation of man's creativity. When you dine in a restaurant you experience the efforts of creative endeavor, from the growing of food to its preparation to its serving. When you use a telephone you experience much more than being able to talk to someone who is separated from you by physical distance. You are using the benefits of others' creative endeavors from Alexander Graham Bell and Nicola Tesla to the local telephone company employees who make your call possible.

To begin conceiving the essence of creative energy is to appreciate its expression in our everyday lives. Most take their own and other's creativity for granted and for this reason settle for much less than they are capable of producing. Bound by habit, they become mentally lazy causing their minds to dwell in the mediocrity of normalcy thus perpetuating the ills of mankind. In truth, it is easier to create than destroy, to love than to hate, to trust than to fear, to evolve than to stagnate. To become free of self-imposed limitations, break free from compulsion by becoming aware of the freedom inherent in your ability to think. Thinking frees you to see, to hear, to feel, to taste, to smell, and most importantly to perceive.

As reasoning is understood and utilized, creativity flourishes. Wherever you experience expressions of man's creativity, you will find the use of creative energy. When this creativity is used by an evolved soul with the highest ideals and purposes in mind, you will find the use of the Kundalini for in this type of expression all of humanity benefits.

In our pursuit of knowledge of Kundalini, it is well that we examine the lives of those possessing expanded awareness. In their thoughts we find the Universal Truth, and Universal Truth can be applied in anyone's life at any time. The thinking of these evolved souls rises above the normal, challenging limitations accepted by the masses, paving the way for advancement for all. Those displaying this expanded consciousness are often described as living before their time. Yet it is their willingness to stimulate others—even in the face of severe opposition—toward the attainment of the visions they conceive that propels them to a place reserved for history's greats. As it has been said, *"Talent does what it can, genius does what it must."* By investigating and putting to use the talent you possess, you can become known for your creativity. By expanding your consciousness to include all of mankind, you can become known for your genius. The creative genius' thinking includes the world and all of humanity, for this reason, in time he is revered and remembered.

Creativity is abundant in man's search for Self expression. From a piece of art that captures the soul to the preparation of a meal that delights the senses, from the ability to explore outer space to the composition of a letter, every day the mind is used for creative endeavors. Yet many are restless in the accepted limitations of complacency. They desire to soar beyond what is considered normal and expand their consciousness to ever evolving states of creativity. By exposing ourselves to the quality of thinking of those remembered in our history as masters of reasoning, we can begin to align our thoughts with our own inner urge to create. What faculties does the individual who comes to be known as a genius possess that elevates his status to that of a master of creativity? What thoughts fill the consciousness of the creative genius?

History is filled with evidence of great thinkers. These individuals have furthered our progress as individuals, as societies, and as a race known as mankind. Their lives are varied. The consequences of birth hold no limitation for these individuals, for we find the complete range—master or slave, rich or poor, educated or not—of experiences represented in their lives. From the early thinkers who learned to harness the four basic elements of air, fire, water, and earth to make physical life easier to more recent thinkers who use the same elements to enhance the mental evolution of man, we find inspiration in the lives of these thinkers. They embody the finest we can become and the wisdom in their thoughts enables us to share their vision of the spiritual unfoldment that is our destiny. To become acquainted with these thinkers is to witness the benefits of the awakening of the Kundalini energy available to man. Their lives are evidence of Kundalini in action for the benefit of all and their conclusions reflect the awareness of a consciousness expanded.

The willingness to extend the boundaries of our thinking is well described in a quote by Oliver Wendell Holmes, Jr.:

*"Man's mind, stretched to a new idea, never
goes back to its original dimension."*

It is true that as we reach for food for thought, just as the legendary woman in the garden of Eden, we become like gods enhancing our awareness of creation. Embracing new ideas strengthens our ability to move beyond limitations no longer dependent upon someone or something outside of ourselves for spiritual salvation, mental guidance, emotional balance, or physical stability.

Holmes was an American jurist born in 1841. A Harvard graduate, he taught law there until he was appointed to the Massachusetts Supreme Court. He believed that law was made for man, not the other way around. Laws were an answer to man's need for cooperative order rather than a body of absolute rules. Theodore Roosevelt appointed him to the U.S. Supreme Court in 1902 where Holmes served for thirty years.

Holmes' observation of the expansion of consciousness is the backbone of individual evolution sparking the rise of Kundalini. By considering, evaluating, and embracing new ways of thinking the progression of the soul is promoted. This continual exercising of creative power and authority precipitates the arousal of Kundalini. Activation of the serpent power demands a change in consciousness. Moving beyond previously accepted limitations, it is the mind in its imaginative glory that is the parent conceiving new ways of thought and life which will culminate in the enlightenment of man.

The founding fathers of the United States knew of esoteric truths since most of them were Freemasons and many were Unitarian in religious thought. They intended the new country to be the first nation in the world founded on the basis of reason. Esoteric meaning shines throughout the symbols, such as the Great Seal, created to represent the new alliance. The notation of "In God We Trust" was an affirmation of their belief that the mind of man reflects the mind of God. They also believed it is reason which puts man in touch with God, and since all people are capable of reason this served as the fundamental principle of democracy. Their creativity reached far beyond its physical manifestations, and they revered the individual's spiritual birthright to excel and progress.

In the original draft of America's Declaration of Independence, Thomas Jefferson wrote:

> *"We hold these truths to be sacred and undeniable; that all men are created equal and independent, that from the equal creation they derive rights inherent and inalienable, among which are preservation of life and liberty, and the pursuit of happiness."*

He is remembered as the third president of the United States, yet Thomas Jefferson expressed his creativity in a variety of ways. He was a lawyer, a farmer, a statesman, a governor, a minister to France, and an architect. He believed his greatest life accomplishment was the founding of a university. It is the expansiveness of his consciousness which qualifies him to be considered a creative genius.

Jefferson's use of physical existence serves as an example of the rewards enjoyed by someone who uses creativity to envision activities based on the highest principles of the good for all. His burning desire to give excellence shows much more in how his creations affected others beyond his own time than in the status and position he attained during his lifetime.

By the time the final draft of the Declaration of Independence was written, Jefferson's words were slightly altered. One change affirmed the Founding Fathers' belief in man's divine nature and is expressed in the phrase *"are endowed by their Creator"*. Far beyond any ideas of conflicts of church and state, the Freemasons who founded our country spoke from what was then occult knowledge of the existence, nature, and purpose of man and his inherent right to become like his Creator.

This was recognized by an outstanding individual over one hundred years after the formation of the United States. A Nobel prize winner who became a U.S. citizen in 1940, Albert

Einstein (1879-1955) once remarked,

*"Making allowances for human imperfections,
I do feel that in America the most valuable thing
in life is possible, the development of the individual and his creative powers."*

An independent, uncompromising thinker, he expressed himself
freely on social, religious, and educational issues. His choice to
change his citizenship from his native Germany was no doubt
influenced by the idea of individual freedom and responsibility
to evolve.

It is true in order for creativity to flourish man must have
the freedom of responsibility for his thoughts and actions. In the
United States, anyone can excel, anyone can dream and with a
directed mind anyone can live that dream. This atmosphere
promotes the development and use of Kundalini energy. Many
believe the awakening of Kundalini can only be gained through
Eastern disciplines, and although a disciplined mind is required
for her use, it is the consistent act of creation which stimulates
the Kundalini.

Native American scientist and inventor, Thomas Alva
Edison (1847-1931) recognized these principles as well. Born
in Milan, Ohio, he had three months of formal education in
Michigan, and at 21 years of age received his first patent for an
electrical vote recorder. In half a century he patented 1033
inventions including the phonograph, the incandescent lamp
with carbon filament, the storage battery, motion picture camera, and the electric railway. It was Edison who said, *"What man's
mind can create, man's character can control."*

In addition to an expansion of consciousness, activated
Kundalini demands an *elevation* of consciousness. The mind
must move beyond concerns for personal physical want, becoming occupied with the needs of all humanity. Such a thinker
continually asks, "How can what I think and do benefit others?"
This expansion of thought causes one to move beyond the
isolation of physical immaturity into the refined awareness of

relativity as the soul seeks to mature. This kind of thinking defines character producing the sustained motivation needed for innovation to develop.

To know your place in creation, to maintain this expanded consciousness when others do not, to respond for someone else's good as readily as you do your own, signifies an opening of consciousness. Lucius Annaeus Seneca described it in this way,

"Most powerful is he who has himself in his own power."

To be able to include others in your thoughts requires Self knowledge, Self direction, and Self possession. Seneca (3 B.C. - 65 A.D.) was born in Spain and educated by Roman Stoics. Appointed tutor to 11 year old Nero, he sought to make him into the ideal philosopher-king. Yet Nero fell prey to what another philosopher four centuries before called a *commoner nature.*

Plato (427-347 B.C.) was a Greek philosopher who established the Academia, scientific training for young men for great public service. The study included mathematics, natural history, practical legislation, and dialectics. The Academia was the first university of its kind, lasting 900 years until it was closed by Justinian in 529 A.D. Aristotle, teacher of Alexander the Great, was a student of Plato. Plato taught the world that ideas or forms alone are real and permanent, while their physical manifestation are merely imperfect copies.

With his metaphysical view of the world, Plato observed and drew many conclusions concerning the type of thought necessary for mankind to progress peacefully. He realized the unification of thought and action in leadership would produce the expansion of consciousness capable of providing peaceful coexistence. In one of his writings, he described this idea in this way:

"Until philosophers are kings, or the kings and princes of this world have the spirit and power of philosophers, and political greatness and wis-

*dom meet in one, and those commoner natures
who pursue either to the exclusion of the other
one compelled to stand aside, cities will never
rest from their evils."*

Centuries later, a well known and loved American described a similar view,

*"God grant that not only the love of liberty but a
thorough knowledge of the rights of man may
pervade all the nations of the earth, so that a
philosopher may set foot anywhere on its surface
and say 'This is my country'."*

Benjamin Franklin (1706-1790) is remembered as a statesman, writer, printer, and inventor. To his credit he founded an academy which became the University of Pennsylvania. He also started a militia, the first fire company, and the first hospital in the colonies. For twenty five years he wrote and published *Poor Richard's Almanac*. He invented the lightning rod, bifocal glasses, the Franklin stove, and the water harmonica. He was deputy postmaster general of the colonies, helped draft the Declaration of Independence, and was ambassador to France. Through his choices, Franklin exemplified the unity of thought and action, philosophy and leadership, described by Plato centuries before. His exceptional use of creativity in an abundance of physical expressions remains an example of one lifetime richly lived in service to anyone, anywhere, at any time. This universal quality is another mark of Kundalini well used for the benefit of humanity.

Also characteristic of the use of Kundalini in the great thinkers of history is their preoccupation with truth. In the Descent of Man, Charles Darwin observed,

*"False facts are highly injurious to the pro-
gression of men, for they often endure long; but
false views, if supported by some evidence, do*

little harm, for everyone takes a salutary plea-
sure in proving their falseness; and when this is
done, one path towards error is closed and the
road to truth is often at the same time opened."

As we reach to understand the universal nature of truth, our consciousness is expanded beyond the limits of individual truth and our creativity is freed to flourish in a world which extends far beyond our own experience.

Charles Darwin (1809-1882) entered Edinburgh at sixteen to study medicine upon the urging of his physician father. Within three years he had left for Cambridge to prepare for the ministry. His interest in natural history increased, and a five year voyage to South America and Australia in the early 1830's began his life long study of flora, fauna, and geology to shed light on the origin of the species. By daring to challenge long held ideas of creation, Darwin like many before him stretched his own thinking beyond what was commonly accepted, and in sharing his discovery dared us to do the same. He allowed his creativity to birth new conclusions which moved his individual perception of truth into the realm of the universal.

A contemporary of Darwin, noted American educator Horace Mann, also realized the importance of pursuing truth. Simply and well stated, Mann described the intention of those remembered as creative geniuses,

"If any man seeks for greatness, let him forget
greatness and ask for truth, and he will find
both."

Horace Mann (1796-1859) was raised in a poor Massachusetts family. Sparsely schooled, he graduated with honors from Brown University with a law degree. Appointed secretary of the Board of Education, he spent twelve years working to improve the state's deteriorated school system in the face of bitter opposition. He increased teaching standards and pay, and improved buildings and equipment. After spending two terms in Congress, he served as president of Antioch College in Ohio which which became a laboratory for his ideas on co-education and nonsectarian education.

No doubt his suggestion for one *"to forget greatness and ask for truth"* was well-earned from personal experience for another indication of Kundalini aroused is the progressive thought precipitating her rise. Such progressive thought always meets with opposition, ridicule, and personal attacks from those consumed by the limitations of a closed, and therefore small, mind. It has been to the retardation of humanity's evolution that these types of limited thinkers are often found not only in our neighbors but also in those who hold respected and powerful positions. It is for this reason that the creative genius of many goes unrecognized until the lifetime has passed and future generations have opened their consciousness to accept the import of those who furthered our evolution through their courage to support the truth they had found even in the face of any opposition.

For a thinker to draw upon the creative power of Kundalini once or twice in a lifetime is commonplace. What sets the creative genius apart from the average man, is the willingness to use her again and again. Johann Wolfgang von Goethe described it in this way,

> *"The chief thing is to have a soul that loves the truth and harbors it where it finds it. And another thing: the truth requires constant repetition, because error is being preached about us all the time, and not only by isolated individuals but by the masses. In newspapers and encyclopedias, in schools and universities, everywhere error rides high and basks in the consciousness of having the majority on its side."*

Goethe was born in Frankfurt. He wrote in several languages and commanded a knowledge of art before he was 10. Studying music, drawing, natural history, and law, he was devoted to alchemy, chemistry, occult philosophy, anatomy, literature, and antiquities. A Chief Minister of State and Director of the State Theater and Scientific Institute, he is best remembered for his great dramatic poem Faust although his Metamorphosis of Plants was a forerunner of Darwin's new theory on light. Goethe sought to make his life an expression of man's complete potential. An inner desire and willingness to seek full development of Self leads to the awakening of the creative energy in Man, and is an attitude shared by those recognized for their genius throughout history.

To be a whole, functioning Self, is to have direct experience with the truths of the universe and to know creation. Confucius said,

> *"Those who know the truth are not equal to those who love it."*

To define personal truth is a forebearer and prerequisite to comprehending truth of a universal nature. Universal Truths apply to anyone, anywhere, and at any time in our universe. Acts of creation produce an awareness of the universal power of love and its transcendent quality. During his life, Confucius (551-479 B.C.) was a government official during a period of corruption, tyranny, and warfare among Chinese states. Seeking change and resolve of conflict, he proposed a code of ethics for the management of society that would unify wisdom and government. His thoughts are recorded in the Analects which remain the tenets for a school of thought known today as Confucianism.

Shortly after Confucius' time, another creative genius Siddhartha Gautama (563-483 B.C.) was born in India. Unlike Confucius, Gautama's experiences led him to renounce his physical birthright and pursue a spiritual calling. A prince at birth, it was prophesied Gautama would become a great ruler or great teacher. At 29, he saw an old man, a sick man, a corpse, and a wandering religious mendicant. The first three revealed to him the suffering in the world, and the tranquility of the fourth suggested his destiny. Gautama is quoted as having said,

*"Though one should in battle conquer a thousand
men a thousand times, he who conquers himself
has the more glorious victory."*

His growing recognition of man's need to achieve a state of
desirelessness led to the renunciation of his heritage and pursuit
of the enlightenment resulting from Self mastery. The expanded
consciousness he attained is attested by the title he bore, Buddha.

Although renunciation of physical pleasure, position,
and possession is not a prerequisite for the use of Kundalini,
consciousness must be altered to include what is unseen by the
physical eye thus developing the perception of Self to include
the parts of Self beyond physical existence. Socrates (469-399
B.C.) was the Athenian son of a sculptor and stonecutter. What
we know of him is because of the writings of his student Plato.
In Apology, Plato records this insight from Socrates,

*"I do nothing but go about persuading you all,
old and young alike, not to take thought for your
persons or your properties, but first to chiefly to
care about the greatest improvement of the soul.
I tell you that virtue does not come from money
but that from virtue comes money and every
other good of man, public as well as private."*

Socrates' instruction was to use the physical existence for
permanent learning which would transcend the physical lifetime
becoming a part of the soul.

When the Kundalini is awakened in man, the recognition
of the transitory nature of the physical produces the realization
of a greater purpose for existence. Guided by the divine voice
of his daemon, Socrates saw his mission as a search for knowledge
which would lead to virtuous living. Pronounced wisest of all
men by the Delphic Oracle, Socrates held that his wisdom came
from his recognition of his own ignorance while others claiming
wisdom were unaware of their ignorance. From this he devel-

oped a method of teaching knowledge by seeking it at the same time. Many creative geniuses have sought to use their creativity to advance the learning of Self while passing on their conclusions to others in either formal or informal instruction. By teaching others, ideas are expanded, conclusions are quickened, and developments are accelerated, while the truth of the knowledge is made a part of the soul.

As this awareness is achieved, the words of a famous Russian author, Fyodor Dostoevsky, ring true,

"Perhaps the only goal on earth toward which mankind is striving lies in the process of attaining, in other words, in life itself, and not in the thing to be attained."

Through his experiences, Dostoevsky realized the Universal Truth of man's destiny as a creator.

Dostoevsky (1821-1881) was the Moscow born son of a tyrannical army surgeon who was murdered by his serfs. Having graduated from military engineering schools in St. Petersburg, he turned to writing. A member of a socialist reading group he was arrested in 1849 and faced a firing squad only to be told his sentence was commuted to hard labor in Siberia. He spent four years among criminals and outcasts which gave him insights into the lowest order of society. The one book permitted him, *The New Testament,* stimulated expansive thinking reflected in the religious mysticism of his later great novels including Crime and Punishment and Brothers Karamazov.

It does not seem to matter when someone exists, or where on earth they are born, or the conditions of their birth. No physical situations are a limit to the innate Spirit of man to progress and evolve. When a developed soul enters a lifetime with purpose and cooperation exists in the consciousness of the physical person as he moves through his lifetime, the potential for genius exists. As demonstrated in the thoughts and deeds of those noted here, any one of us has the potential for the creativity that produces the enlightenment they embody.

As Victor Marie Hugo (1802-1885), the author of Hunchback of Notre Dame and Les Miserables said,

"Nothing else in the world...is so powerful as an idea whose time has come."

Hugo grew up during the Napoleonic era. At four he wrote his first tragedy, at twenty his first book. He revolutionized the rigid forms of poetry, and mixed tragedy and comedy in his dramas. In addition to using writing as an expression of creativity, Hugo was involved in governmental leadership as a senator in the third republic of France.

The great thinkers quoted here stand with many others who have advanced humanity with their vision of what can be. By creating their thoughts with the highest ideal and purpose, they transformed greed into ambition and the entire world has benefited from their drive to excel and make a better world. Their lives are testimonies of creativity directed toward physical accomplishment. Their thoughts confirm the use of creativity in non-physical endeavors. Transcending physical structures and boundaries, the thinking worthy of a creative genius shines through the words of these men attesting to the birth of Spiritual enlightenment characteristic of the use of Kundalini. They serve as examples to be emulated. Their thoughts ignite an inner urge toward creative genius in anyone willing to open his mind. The Truths they discovered, shared, and endeavored to live stimulate the deepest and highest thoughts we can perceive.

For those who have awakened to man's challenge to mature as a creator, Kundalini beckons. It is time for man to rise from a sleeping consciousness of the common, the norm, the habitual. More and more, people are restless, attempting to stir from lifetimes of Self repression and deceit. People are ready to open their eyes to the wonders of Self mastery and enlightenment. *"Nothing else in the world...is so powerful as an idea whose time has come."* The time to embrace the idea of Kundalini rising has indeed arrived for us all.

Sleeping Consciousness

The evidence of Kundalini rising in man lies in his evolving consciousness. Man's need to know Self as a Spiritual being beyond his finite material existence wells up from within him. This dynamic inner urge for spiritual growth is ever-present, seeking to reveal itself to a sleeping consciousness.

For most, the senses have an attractive power acting like magnets consistently drawing the mind's attention to the physical world and holding the thinker earthbound. When this occurs man looks for security to come from his physical situations and circumstances thus becoming a slave to his physical experiences. Rather than examining our own thoughts which lead to differences in opinion, beliefs, and lifestyle, we will accuse, ridicule, and wage war on those who oppose us. Rather than use creative thinking to correct mistakes in judgement, we will blindly and compulsively enter into new situations with the same attitudes as before thus enduring similar unpleasant and undesirable experiences. Rather than developing inwardly through inner mind communication commonly called dreams, we relish the opportunity to lose consciousness in hours of sleep. Rather than seek guidance from our inner divinity through meditation to expand understanding, we call upon a higher power existing outside of ourselves to mysteriously heal our pain. Every moment we possess the opportunity for greater Self awareness, yet most

forfeit this innate right to choose producing a sleeping consciousness, entrapped by the limitations of the physical existence
and inattentive to potential enlightenment.

Sleeping consciousness results from dependency upon
the physical alone as a means of Self identity. When you allow
your sense of who you are to be dictated by the conditions in your
physical life only, your consciousness is lulled into a deceptive
state of peace and turbulence which is temporary. Your awareness
of existence beyond the physical conditions in your life escapes
recognition and you are buffeted by those conditions which exist
only momentarily. One day you may be the highest paid
executive in your firm, the next day you may find yourself
unemployed. One day you may lose your spouse through
divorce or death, and another day you may find your closest
friend to be the "soulmate" you have been seeking. One day you
may have one dollar, and another day multiply this thousands of
times. One day you may be a parent, and another day be
childless. One day you may move into the house of your dreams,
and another day see that house disappear through natural disaster
or mismanagement of funds. One day you may receive a medical
"death sentence", and another day become a medical "miracle".

Since the nature of the physical is change, the conditions
in your life are constantly in motion. When your identity is
solely formed from a physical position in life, the consciousness
of who you are is severely limited. You can experience the
elation, pride, and security produced by being outstanding in a
career, in love, as a parent, as an owner of a house, or in robust
health, and you can also experience the confusion, frustration,
and depression produced from the lack of these desired conditions. When there is a willingness to expand thinking beyond
the physical situations in life, you cause your consciousness to
awaken to who you are. Being an executive, a spouse, a parent,
the owner of possessions, even being healthy are temporary
physical conditions. Their longevity is limited to a single
lifetime. Who you really are expands far beyond these physical
limitations. It is this Real Self which the Kundalini beckons you
to admit, explore, and experience.

In the play *Hamlet*, William Shakespeare describes man in this way:

What a piece of work is man! how noble in reason! how infinite in faculties! in form and moving how express and admirable! in action how like an angel! in apprehension how like a god! the beauty of the world! the paragon of animals!

Aptly described through the creative genius of Shakespeare is the essence of our ability to transcend the limitations of the physical and our animal bodies. One of the most dynamic differences between man and animals is the potential to experience, understand, and direct the use of the Kundalini. Although Kundalini exists in all life forms, man uses the only form sufficiently evolved to wield her creative power. The highly developed vehicle of the physical body and brain gives us the necessary equipment for voluntary spiritual evolution. The cerebral cortex of the brain, the juxtapositioning of the thumb and fingers, and the tailless vertebral column distinguish man's body from all other animals. It also enables him to use highly developed thinking abilities not found in other planetary life forms. This causes us to rise above instinct and compulsion evidenced in earlier life forms through the use of conscious reasoning.

The availability of reasoning, including the faculties of memory, attention, and imagination, gives us the power to perceive and with perception comes the awakening of consciousness. Once awakened, we can move and live and breathe in dimensions of inner consciousness beyond the physical and unlock the creative potential worthy of being an offspring of a Creator.

The inner urge for this expansion of consciousness often makes itself known through spontaneous bursts of Kundalini energy. For some this can be interpreted as a sense of urgency that arises from no apparent cause. As the energy becomes active in consciousness, you may find new thoughts running through your mind. "Shouldn't I be doing something better with my life" or "There must be a purpose for my existence".

Years ago while attending college at the University of Missouri, two friends and I were making plans to leave the confines of dormitory life and make a new home in an apartment off-campus. My life was filled with expectation and excitement about the prospective move. My relationships were fulfilling and I was proving to be successful in my educational endeavors looking forward to the challenges of a career upon graduation. I was "doing what I was supposed to be doing" with only momentary lapses of thought into the reason for it all.

Coming from visiting the place we would soon call home, we were in a car accident involving our car and two others. I was driving the car we were riding in, and at the moment of collision I saw the chain of events as though I was riding in a helicopter above the scene. My body remained in the car, instinctively controlling its movement, but the point of reference for my consciousness was from a point several hundred feet in the air looking down. I could see my tan car, the blue car I hit, and the maroon sports car the blue car hit. Once my car ceased motion, my consciousness returned to my body and I was fully aware of being behind the steering wheel again.

My thoughts raced. The first thoughts were of over-whelming responsibility. My friends went to check on the other drivers, returning with reports of their conditions. Amidst the disorientation of the first few minutes following the accident, my mind quickly moved from denial and a weak-willed wish that this had not occurred to a fervent plea for assistance from a power greater than my own for the safety of all involved which later was fulfilled. Yet at the time I wondered why I and my friends were not hurt and the other drivers experienced cuts and bruises. I wrestled with the misuse of freedom I had demonstrated. I had abused my reputation as a safe and careful driver. What was now occurring was because of my failed awareness of responsibility. Amidst my thoughts of condemnation, I vowed to make concentrated efforts to heal my shattered confidence in being able to responsibly control a motor vehicle.

Once these lessons were learned, my consciousness began to open. Repeatedly, the question "Why?" filled my mind. Why did it happen? I had never caused an accident. I did have a reputation as a safe driver. Why did I choose this route to return instead of another? If I'd chosen another route, this accident would not have happened. Why now, when everything in my life was moving forward? Why were my friends with me when it happened? Why couldn't I have been alone and spared them potential harm? Why were two other cars involved? Why were we unscarred, and the other drivers hurt? Why wasn't I hurt instead of the others? My consciousness had been expanded.

In all the why's that surfaced from my inner thoughts, beyond all surface considerations of denial, guilt, blame, and fear, an overwhelming realization became clearly apparent. Faced with a very real physical situation that could have resulted in my causing someone serious injury or death, and faced with my own mortality, my consciousness was expanded to include my inner urge to know my reason for existence. Without doubt I knew my life had been spared for a reason, and I admitted that I did not yet know what that reason was. At the time I had only metaphysical questions which had suddenly moved from the periphery of my consciousness to the center of my conscious being. Issues I previously dismissed or pushed aside, now refused to disappear in a fog of denial. My consciousness now included a sense of urgency for finding answers that would be logically sound, universally applicable, and personally revelatory. The sense of urgency produced by the seemingly unanswerable is a precursor of Kundalini aroused.

Others have experienced this arousal as a result of near-death experiences. Documented cases abound in recent years of out-of-body experiences leading to the recognition of existence beyond the physical plane. Some report observing the body being attended by medical professionals while the consciousness gives the perspective of an observer to the physical scene. Following this experience, patients report comments made or physical details of others' actions to the amazement of those present who believed the patient was sedated and unaware of events transpiring. For someone entrapped in the body alone, he would remain unconscious of such events, but to one who has moved beyond the limitations of the physical such knowledge can be made a part of consciousness. Spontaneous out-of-body experiences are characteristic of the arousal of Kundalini.

Others experiencing near-death conditions have reported moving through a tunnel toward a light. Many times friends or relatives who have already died appear, offering what is perceived as comfort, encouragement, or counsel. Actress Elizabeth Taylor tells of a near death experience where she passed through a tunnel toward a light. There she met Mike Todd, her former husband who had been killed in a plane wreck. She reports that Mike told her she had to go back, that it was not yet time for her to stay. Returning back to physical life, Elizabeth has continued to live many years of a life rich in experience. She has spoken of her near-death experience as impressive because it freed her from any fear of physical death.

Greeting those who have previously ceased physical existence is a common occurrence in near-death experiences. Because the consciousness has passed physical boundaries of sensory experience, the individual finds his awareness extended into the inner levels of consciousness where these entities reside. In essence, the movement of consciousness enables the person to communicate with others who no longer possess a physical body. This communication is from spirit to spirit and it produces an awareness of the continuity of existence. Much more than wish fulfillment, the interchanges between the person nearing physical death and those who have already relinquished physical life are comparable to a conversation you might have today with a loved one. Each display independent thought often offering surprising revelation and unexpected ideas.

Several years ago, my grandmother came to me during a night time dream experience. Having recorded and studied my dreams for many years, I had learned how to detect the difference between messages from my inner, subconscious mind, and actual experiences in the inner levels of consciousness. When I had returned fully to physical consciousness I was puzzled by this visitation. I wondered why my grandmother had sought me out and why she had asked of me the metaphysically oriented questions during our inner level communion. Two days later I received a telephone call from my father informing me that my grandmother had passed away in her sleep the night before. Immediately I remembered our experience and understood why she had come to me. She was preparing to withdraw her consciousness from the physical and had reached out to me for support and guidance.

During the funeral I perceived my grandmother's presence. We telepathically communicated and I knew she was at peace, experiencing the heavenly state she had always believed existed while she was alive in the physical. When my grandfather could no longer contain his grief, I shared my experience of telepathic communication with her. Although it did little to remove his sorrow of loss, it did give him comfort and strength in the knowledge that her soul was a peace and it gave him hope in his ability to reach a state of awareness that could lead to his own direct communication with her.

Many experience clear and vivid night time dreams as a result of spontaneous awakening of Kundalini. These messages from the inner Self become progressively prolific, enabling the dreamer to fill pages with a record of his inner life. Those dream experiences often prove to be precognitive, giving the dreamer prior knowledge of events occurring in his own life or that of others.

To acknowledge our existence beyond the five physical senses is the beginning of awakening our consciousness from the temporary sleep of a physical lifetime. More and more mankind's thinking is moving beyond barriers of previously accepted ways of thinking. A recent Gallup survey in the United States testifies to this expansion of consciousness. The poll revealed:

- *One of every four Americans believes in life after death.*
- *One in ten claims to have seen or been in the presence*

of a "ghost".
* *One in six Americans has felt he has been in touch with someone who has died.*
* *One of every four Americans believes he has had a telepathic experience in which he communicated with another person without using the traditional five senses.*

The expansion of consciousness begins with the consideration of "what if" which precipitates new ideas and belief concepts. Through a scientific approach to investigation, study and research, believing evolves into the knowing gained only through personal, direct experience. In the time and space between believing and knowing lies unlimited possibilities for the use of Kundalini to accelerate the individual's recognition of reality and truth.

Most who return to physical consciousness following a near-death experience, an out-of-body experience, or even profound dream states, birth deeper insights into the purpose for physical existence. Having expanded their consciousness into the realms existing beyond the limits of the physical, their concepts of life become more open and embracing. Many describe this raison d'etre as giving love or sharing love with others. Composer Amadeus Wolfgang Mozart said, "*Neither a lofty degree of intelligence nor imagination nor both together go to the making of genius. Love that is the soul of genius.*" This expansion of consciousness produces a peace and motivation that results from the activation of Kundalini.

Many times the arousal of Kundalini can be the result of religious devotion. One of the best examples of this is seen through the experience of faith healing. Whether described as the power of God or the indomitable human spirit, a profound belief in goodness or wholeness can cause the spontaneous release of Kundalini energy producing immediate physical effects. Cataracts disappear. Kidney stones are passed. Alcohol or drug addictions are broken. Depression or mental disorientation is healed. Although scientists and medical professionals can debate the cause for such occurrences, the fact remains that people continue to experience extreme and immediate cures without the assistance of modern technology. Admitting the creative power in man rather than discounting it frees us to investigate the limitlessness of consciousness which has produced technological advances. It allows for the use of the benefits of creativity without prejudice concerning how the benefits are derived. When this occurs we are no longer a slave to our creativity, rather we move toward the mastery awakened consciousness affords.

Often linked to religious fervor but by no means limited to it, the sense of having a mission, a purpose, a duty, or a calling is also a mark of the arousal of Kundalini. English statesman William E. Gladstone (1809-1898) said that duty is *"a power that rises with us in the morning, and goes to rest with us at night. It is co-extensive with the action of our intelligence. It is the shadow that cleaves to us, go where we will."* George Washington, the first president of the United States, also experienced this sense of purpose noting, *"The consideration that human happiness and moral duty are inseparably connected, will always continue to prompt me to promote the former by inculcating the practice of the latter."* French essayist Michel E. Montaigne extended their sentiment to all thinkers when he wrote: *"Know thyself and do thine own work, says Plato; and each includes the others and covers the whole duty of man."*

When you can ask yourself "Shouldn't I be doing something better with my life" and creatively answer yourself with a vision of who you are and what you can offer the world, you have experienced an expansion of consciousness. The sense of being in the world to accomplish is an important part of the consciousness of anyone who shapes the destiny of the multitudes. You will find it present in world leaders, leading scientists, great artists, and innovative thinkers throughout history. The sense of Self importance combined with a desire to aid others is a mark of a consciousness illumined.

As has been true throughout history, pursuing your own awareness of duty does not always meet with support and recognition even by your closest of friends. Again and again historical figures have met with extreme opposition, sometimes even imprisonment and death at the hands of those filled with fear and threat for their own beliefs and positions. The lives of Galileo Galilei, Christopher Columbus, Jesus of Nazareth, Mohandas K. Gandhi, Martin Luther King, Jr., and countless others attest to this. Unfortunately, ridicule is still a part of human nature, but as people like us endeavor to know and manifest our own sense of duty the world becomes a more receptive place for creative minds to be nurtured and blossom.

Having reached this point in our evolution, most are conscious of a desire to make the world a better place to live. When consciousness moves beyond "why doesn't someone do something" or "why can't he or she do it this way", to "what can I do to improve the quality of life" then the Kundalini has become activated. For many, this arousal does not take place until they produce and bear children. The experience of male and female coming together to produce offspring is much more than a biological occasion. It is a use of Kundalini energy channeled toward physical procreation. Because man has volition, every step of the physically animalistic ritual is a matter of choice. We choose our mate. We choose intercourse. We can even choose the time and sex of our creation. If we cannot easily produce our own offspring, we can choose to adopt another's as our own. Man has volition which gives him the freedom to create in ways that set him apart from the rest of creation. The availability for creating is omnipresent and when one learns to cause the Kundalini energy to rise up the spine to the brain centers inner creation is experienced. The awareness with which you respond to your potential will determine if and how the Kundalini is activated in your consciousness.

Many new parents are overcome with a sense of humility and awe in their ability to create. Being able to experience the new child with their five senses begets a plethora of mind-expanding thoughts about Self, others, and the world we inhabit. Attitudes of unconditional love, protectiveness, and security are birthed and mingled with hopes for stability, peace, prosperity, and health. By creating and experiencing the manifestation of that creation, awareness grows and the desire to better the world can move from the realm of criticizing others to the duty of personal responsibility. Realizing the world is as you make it, knowing your influence can make a difference for others, and becoming a visionary leader is also a result of expanded consciousness. For one who has experienced this arousal of Kundalini, the world becomes your neighbor because you know the relativity of all mankind.

More and more public awareness is growing in the realization that as we progress as a society we are responsible for our creations. Evidence of this awakening of consciousness is perhaps most profoundly demonstrated in the evolution of ecology consciousness. We are becoming aware that our man made creations -- from disposal baby diapers to the harnessing of nuclear energy -- designed for convenience and physical ease or comfort may become the source of future inconvenience, difficulty, and disease.

Some display precognition in their thinking. They are willing to look before they leap into new creative endeavors whose future effects will harm our environment and life on the planet. They impress the need for change now in corporate structures and products. They put themselves on the line by bringing to the masses' attention the need for responsible choices to insure a positive future for ourselves and our posterity. These individuals are leaders in thought, not always popular with a complacent and passive populace who has become accustomed to the instant benefits of someone else's creative genius. They serve as a conscience for us all.

Ecology is one way man is trying to consciously respond to the fact that he is a creator for in creating he has produced not only wonderful conveniences but also a multitude of waste from those creations. It is becoming more apparent that something needs to change so energy is not wasted, but made useful. As sleeping consciousness awakens we discover we live in a wholistic world. Our actions of today produce the situations in our lives tomorrow. What you may have learned as "one man's garbage is another man's treasure" is a truth we can all live by to create a more productive world.

It is true that as a society we are negligent by our shortsightedness. For instance, we annually throw away enough office and writing paper to build a wall twelve feet high stretching from Los Angeles to New York City. Every year we dispose of twenty four million tons of leaves and grass clippings we could have recycled for the nutrients. The United States leads the world in the generation of trash. We average 3.5 to 5 pounds of trash per person per day. The average family produces 100 pounds of trash per week. Every winter the energy equivalent of all the oil that flows through the Alaskan pipeline in a year leaks through American windows. Los Angeles residents drive 142 million miles every day, the distance from Earth to Mars. Astounding isn't it?

There have been recycling efforts that have been established in the last several years. For instance, the energy saved from one recycled aluminum can will operate a television for three hours. In 1988 alone, aluminum can recycling saved more than 11 billion kilowatt hours of electricity which supplies the residential needs of New York City for six months.

How do you measure up in terms of physical ecology? Are you part of the solution, or part of the problem? Are you a leader in change, or are you ignoring the issue thinking its somebody else's problem or someone else's cause? Those with awakened consciousness are concerned. They are not above admitting a problem and initiating change in order to live life more fully.

Opportunities abound to use physical energy more completely. For instance, stop using disposable plates, cups, and utensils. Sure it may take time to hand wash china or silverware, but you will insure a cleaner environment as well as clean dinnerware. Use rags instead of paper, rags can be washed and reused, an efficient use of energy. Use both sides of a piece of paper when possible, indeed more is not always better. Compose food waste and yard debris, perpetuate the natural cycles of creation. What is waste to a human, can be food for animals or the earth. Let your fingers do the walking, call ahead. Instead of traveling all over town trying to locate a desired object, productively use the convenience of your telephone. Hang out your clothes to dry, learn to cooperate with the elements using natural sources of energy that are FREE! Stop wasting water, make sure you are making use of the water when you turn it on. Don't use electrical appliances for things you can do by hand. There is a great deal of learning and art that can be developed when you craft something with your hands. It awakens your consciousness and unlocks the creative genius within you.

When consciousness sleeps, it is easy to devalue your individual importance. You might think, "It really doesn't matter if I do these things." You must arouse your sleeping consciousness! When you think of all the people you know whom you can influence by your more efficient use of energy, your actions can multiply very quickly. You can make a significant difference because you becomes *we*. As the *we* grows, we can awaken the consciousness of humanity across the planet.

To many, ecology is physical only. It entails working with the physical effects of what we have created. To one with awakened consciousness, it is something much more than this. Ecology is truly universal. The one whose consciousness has awakened seeks to know what energy is and how it can be most effectively used in harmony with the laws of the universe. He or she knows that the universe is animated by energy and its perpetual motion relies upon the constant exchange of energies both manifested and unmanifested. This realization feeds the curiosity of awakened consciousness and fuels the desire to know more about the energy of consciousness, the internal ecology of the Whole Self.

The inner urge to cause energy to move forward so that soul progression can occur is also a sign of awakened consciousness. When you look for ways to do something better, when you begin your day with open curiosity and goodwill, when you stretch your mental muscles, your creative thoughts prepare your consciousness for the arousal of Kundalini. Being willing to experiment in life, combining elements to create something different causes forward motion and opens the door to evolution. All great inventors have exhibited this ability. From Franklin and his kite experiments to the Wright brothers and their flying machine, creative thinkers share a courage that lifts them above the ridicule of limited minds and propels them into the annals of history.

Your urge toward inventiveness may not find its way into history books and legends, yet by respecting who you are and knowing how to respond to your own creative urges you can accelerate the progression of your soul and free your consciousness to experience transcendent bliss. The advances you are willing to make in your life will influence the lives of everyone you touch. In this way, all of humanity benefits from the efforts of the one.

The awakening of consciousness is a personal and singular endeavor. By pursuing spiritual enlightenment with the same resolve you offer your career, your marriage and children, your money and possessions, your health, or anything you value in your physical existence, you will find many doors opening to you for a more rewarding existence. Knowledge of the nature of consciousness can serve to aid you in moving beyond spontaneous bursts of creative energy and lead you to understand and respond to the arousal of Kundalini.

Creative Imagery

Once your consciousness has awakened and you are willing to expand your thinking, new worlds of thought open to you. Creative thinking paves the way for the arousal of your Kundalini energy. This thinking separates man from all other forms of life for only man exhibits the ability for Self awareness and expansion of consciousness. Creative thinking is characterized by familiarity of the existence of Self beyond the physical. To add to your understanding of your meta-physical being, let us investigate man's existence as creative mind.

Our physical world is filled with the manifestations of the creative mind. From the stars we see in the nighttime skies to the music we hear, from the food we taste to the flowers we smell, from the materials we touch to the ideas we communicate, the world around us provides multiple stimulation to our senses. The five physical senses of seeing, hearing, tasting, smelling, and touching enable us to constantly receive information. What we think about the information received and how we choose to respond or react to that information is a matter of perception, the sixth sense. It is developed perception that causes the Kundalini to be called into action in our lives.

To understand perception and its relationship to creativity, let us explore the nature of consciousness. Every moment of every day our physical bodies are surrounded by stimuli. Clocks ticking, television images, car exhaust, soft blankets, fresh rain, each can involve the use of all five senses but often it is one sense which is noted thus drawing the attention of the thinker. The sound of a grandfather clock ticking stimulates us to explore the clock with the other senses. We can see its structure; touch the grain of the wood, smelling its aroma. We can even taste it.

Have you seen a child explore his environment? He will gaze with rapt attention, he will reach to hold the object of his interest. He will smell it, hear it, and often to the dismay of a parent, put the object in his mouth! By using every sense, the child learns to identify what is in his environment, storing this information in the brain for use from that time forward. In this way, memory is created. When memory is combined with attention and imagination, the power in the conscious part of our mind, reasoning, is awakened. Knowledge of this power gives us freedom to create our desires through the process known as visualization.

In today's world, many people are aware of and use visualization. Visualization can be used to produce outstanding works of art, to advance science and technology, and to repair physical bodies that are diseased, yet sometimes it seems to fail. Many call upon the power of visualization without knowing how and why it works. This leaves the mind in a state of belief only, bringing inconsistent results. Sometimes visualization works, sometimes it doesn't. Yet, in truth, visualization always produces according to what is being imaged in the mind of its creator. By gaining information concerning how the mind images, you develop visualization as a mental discipline and skill.

Just as nighttime dreams are more than entertaining images, daydreams are more than pictures created as a means of escaping boredom and the pressures of daily living. By learning to control our daydreams, we learn to put our thoughts into directive action drawing upon more of our mind's power. By using will we select the images we desire to communicate to our inner mind for reproduction. With repeated practice we can hone our creativity into a skill worthy of the potential genius within. By effectively using conscious thinking we expand our consciousness to include more of the whole Self.

By knowing the universal structure of mind, we can better understand the mechanics of its creative power. For any thinker who has achieved the evolutionary stage of reasoning, the individualized intelligence of Self finds its expression through what we will call mind. The mind can be divided into three major divisions each with a particular function and duty. Beginning with the farthest extension of mind from its source, the conscious mind is the part of Self most people are accustomed to using. The conscious mind uses the information stored in its computer, the physical brain, for daily experiencing. Information received through the five physical senses is recorded in the brain for future use. In the early years of childhood, we are taught to identify the vibrations of our physical environment. We learn to distinguish sights, sounds, smells, tastes, and feelings, giving them names for easy identification. In this way we can distinguish red from green or shrill high tones from low bass ones. The opinions we form of what is received is a function of the conscious mind. For instance, we might like wearing green because it is calming whereas red is abrasive, making us stand out in a crowd when we would rather be inconspicuous, or we find shrill, high notes nerve-racking reminding us of screams whereas low, bass tones are perceived as soothing or sexually arousing.

The separation of the information received through the senses and what we think about this information is an important step for unlocking our creative potential for in this way we can distinguish the separation of mind and body, the creator from his creation. The conscious mind finds its power in the ability to reason. With the faculties of memory, attention, and imagination, the conscious mind can move beyond instinct. It is free to choose new experiences or repeat the same ones. With creative thinking, the conscious mind is free to initiate experience with purpose and on purpose. The ability to image ideals and purposes for actions is one mark of creative genius. A creator does not wait for experience to happen, he or she initiates

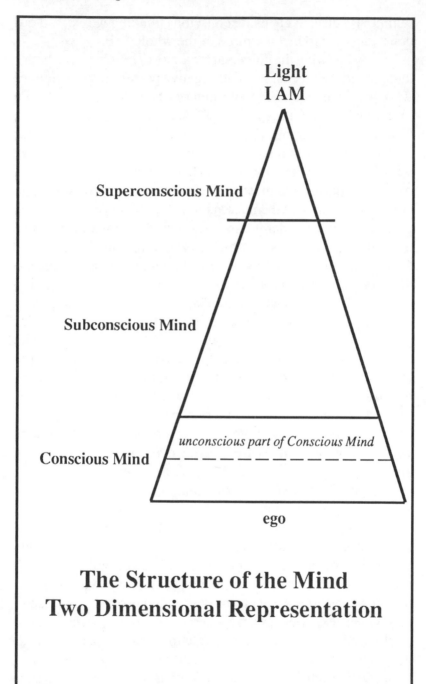

Light
I AM

Superconscious Mind

Subconscious Mind

unconscious part of Conscious Mind

Conscious Mind

ego

The Structure of the Mind
Two Dimensional Representation

experience with intention. When there is awareness of Self identity in the conscious mind, the thinker creates and accelerates his learning and growth throughout a lifetime. The duty of any conscious mind is to gain experiences for the purpose of enhancing the understandings that will become a permanent part of the Self. These understandings then become a part of the inner mind known as the subconscious mind.

The subconscious mind exists beyond the limits of the physical plane of existence. Its power is most aptly described as intuition. While the conscious mind is unconscious during sleep, the subconscious mind offers communication concerning the conscious state of awareness in the form of dreams. The ability for experiencing physically distant places while the physical body remains stationary, known as astral travel or astral projection, is a subconscious mind function. The transference of thoughts from one person to another over long physical distances without the aid of a physical device is known as telepathy, a subconscious mind ability. Clairvoyance, the ability to transcend what the physical eyes alone can see and "see" with the mind, and clairaudience, the ability to transcend the limitations of physical hearing and "listen" with the mind, can be developed through use of the subconscious mind. These and other sixth sense capabilities are natural functions of the subconscious mind. For many they remain shrouded in superstition from lack of investigation and education. Throughout the ages, the subconscious mind has often been referred to in literature as the soul of man. When we are willing to explore and develop Self beyond the limitations of the five physical senses, we begin to move beyond spontaneous bursts of insight, intuition, and creativity. We become cognizant of our soul and are able to draw upon its storehouse of understanding at will. This promotes mastery of creativity.

For most, the realm of subconscious experience remains unconscious. Until this experience is embraced by awareness in the conscious mind, we are ignorant of its function or even its existence. Ignorance, however, does not in any way diminish the importance of the inner Self or destroy its existence. By disciplining and learning to still the conscious mind, we enable our awareness to include this inner part of Self. In this way, what had been unconscious in our conscious mind becomes part of our conscious awareness. For creativity to flourish, this knowledge must become a part of our waking consciousness.

In addition to intuitive faculties, the subconscious part of mind plays an important role in the manifestation of our desires. Its function is to reproduce what the conscious mind desires. In this way, the subconscious mind facilitates the manifestation of experiences and increases the opportunities for greater understanding to be gained by the conscious mind. This enables the subconscious mind to fulfill its duty of housing the understandings that will strengthen the Self's identity as a creator. As the subconscious mind executes its purpose, the Self evolves through lifetimes of physical experiencing. Understandings become more prosperous and a child prodigy is born, affinity for particular means of expression become apparent with little or no external instruction, and another genius shares the benefit of lifetimes of understanding with the world.

The innermost part of the mind can be described as the superconscious mind. Its function is to hold the plan for Self's development as a creator worthy of its Spiritual parental heritage. For this reason, here is where we find inner authority and knowledge of man's divinity. The superconscious mind's duty is to continue to give life to the outer parts of mind as long as it takes the Self to realize its wholeness and achieve enlightenment. As we become more creative, causing the Kundalini energy to rise, a commitment to honor and revere this part of Self must be made a part of our conscious awareness. This commitment is revealed and practiced through daily communion and will be discussed in later chapters.

Understanding the inner workings of visualization frees us for greater creative endeavors. Visualization is both an art and a science, and it can be studied, learned, and refined by its practitioner. Visualization employs an efficient use of the conscious mind and the subconscious mind. By understanding how an imaged thought becomes a physical manifestation, we eliminate many questions and related doubts concerning our ability for effective visualization.

Briefly, when the conscious mind initiates visualization, a sequence of events takes place resulting in the manifestation of what is desired. First, a stimulus is received by the conscious mind. This causes a need to become apparent in our thinking, which we then develop into a desire for something that will fill this need. The contemplation of this results in the production of a thought and creation of a desire-image. By building awareness of our desire-image we call into action the re-creative ability of our subconscious mind setting into motion the inner workings of the visualization process.

For instance, you awake in the morning to the smell of bacon frying. Through the olfactory system of your body, the odor produced is received through sensory nerves until it reaches the pituitary gland in your brain. The pituitary gland is an interpreter of energies. Your pituitary interprets the energy based upon the information you have previously stored in your brain concerning the experience of bacon. Most likely, the interpretation will first stimulate your need for food to nourish your body. If further information is stored in your brain indicating the eating of bacon is a pleasurable experience, a desire for the bacon will be developed in your conscious mind. If further information indicates a distaste for bacon, the visualization process will cease, you will either turn over and go back to sleep, open a window to remove the offensive odor, or find a related food substance you do want to fill your physical need for food.

If you like bacon, you will begin remembering pleasurable eating experiences perhaps going far beyond the taste of bacon and reaching into comforting thoughts of home cooked meals and loving conversations. You will begin to imagine similar conditions when you are able to experience the bacon with all of your senses, when you can see it, taste it, hear it, and touch it as well as smell it. You propel yourself out of bed taking the necessary action to fulfill your developed desire to partake in the morning meal. This simple example describes the step by step process of thinking necessary for visualization to occur. These same steps will be employed to produce any creative experience.

Receptivity to a stimulus is an important first step to unlocking our creativity for it initiates our use of visualization. An open mind, constantly seeking learning, finds stimuli are received in mind-to-mind communication as well as through the five physical senses. This telepathic connection can explain how innovative thinkers separated by thousands of physical miles, unaware of the other's existence, can arrive at similar conclusions at the same time. It is also the reason why that person we have known for years, the one we have worked with day in and day out, suddenly becomes the object of our affection, the man or woman of our dreams. The conscious mind must be open to stimulation for our needs and desires to become apparent. When the mind is closed we live lives of repetitive boredom, shutting out the world around us, ignoring the stimuli that abound, and denying our needs and desires. We end up eating, sleeping, following the leader and eventually dying. A lifetime of promise and opportunity is wasted. When creativity remains stifled by a closed mind, it is little wonder that anger, hatred, sadness, and frustration fills the world.

To be receptive to what life has to offer, is the birth of creativity. By embracing experience, we give our minds food for thought, and by feeding our mind we find resources readily available for our creative endeavors. The company our mind keeps tells us a great deal about ourselves. The way we spend our waking time reveals the state of our awareness and preparedness for expanded consciousness. Once a stimulus is received, we always have the final decision of how we will respond. A ringing telephone is just that, a ringing telephone. We choose our response to it. We decide to answer the call, let a machine answer for us, or to let it keep ringing. Being receptive does not eliminate choice, it heightens it. We become aware of the many avenues open to us. The quality of our choices reflects the nature of our consciousness thus we are attracted by the announcement of a concert by a virtuoso or attracted by an offer to indulge in mind-altering drugs as a means of escaping from a world we do not understand. Only by being willing to receive the stimulus do we have the advantage of determining what our response will be.

Many inventive people seek newness without knowing why. They look for new places to visit, move frequently, eat different foods, enjoy opportunities to make new friends, study different cultures. The advantage of being willing to seek newness is the freshness it affords. Newness demands sensory attentiveness. New places fill our senses with new sights and sounds, new foods stimulate new tastes and smells, new friends and cultures give us a chance to receive new ideas and ways of thinking. Newness is an excellent way to open a closed mind for it gives us the opportunity to be new as well. When you are among strangers, they hold fewer preconceived ideas of who you are.

A willingness toward newness brings with it an attitude of embracing change. The more adaptable we can become, the easier it is for consciousness to expand. Yet, the development of genius also necessitates an openness to perceiving the new in the old. When you can, after years of knowing someone, still discover newness in your relationship with them you have caused a further evolution in your own consciousness. You have achieved an open-mindedness which leads to greater understanding of who you are and of life itself.

By keeping an open and receptive conscious mind, you can be stimulated anytime, anywhere, and with anyone. This frees you to accelerate your learning and soul progression for you are no longer dependent upon any set physical condition of a person, a place, or a thing to stimulate your creativity. You can create anywhere, any place, any time. And this is the mark of a creator.

Once a stimulus is received by the conscious mind, a need will become apparent. In the earlier example, the need to eat was acknowledged. Physical needs of eating, bathing, having shelter, being sufficiently warm, are often taken for granted because we learn them quickly as a means for physical survival. Yet many needs for Reasoning Man exist in the realm of thought. We need communication with other minds, we need to give and receive love and respect, we need a sense of purposefulness in our existence, we need to feel challenged and that we are accomplishing something in our lives. Constantly stimuli surround us beckoning our consciousness to awaken and become aware of our own multi-dimensional needs.

Watching a movie may stimulate our own need for Self expression. Interacting with a new boss may stimulate our need for respect and authority. Being asked questions by a child may stimulate our need for more information or deeper thought. Forgetting someone's name may stimulate our need to develop memory. Losing track of a conversation may stimulate our need for better listening. A nightmare may stimulate our need to understand the meaning of our dreams.

By being aware of what need is being stimulated, we can learn to redirect any limiting emotional reaction to stimuli and admit our desires. Emotional reactions to stimuli steal from our ability to use reasoning in the conscious mind. They distract our attention from our needs and desires, causing us to remain unchanged and at the mercy of our own misunderstandings. Instead of becoming distracted by thoughts of jealousy concerning the actors in the movie, we can admit our desire to entertain and perform. Instead of rebelling against our new boss's authority, we can admit our desire for more responsibility and prestige. Instead of ridiculing the child for asking such questions, we can pursue our desire for answers. Instead of offering a weak apology for forgetting someone's name or failing to listen, we can admit our desire to pay closer attention to situations in our lives. Instead of dismissing nightmares as trivia, we can admit our desire to understand the meaning of this inner communication.

When we allow ourselves to live in jealousy, rebellion, ridicule, apology, and trivia, we weaken our ability to recognize and use our full potential. We foster sleeping consciousness, defining our existence by habitual reactions fueled by a lack of initiative and will power. The initiative to create is known to anyone with an open mind. The development of will power is known to anyone who realizes the importance of their need to progress, to be better today than yesterday. By admitting our needs and identifying desires to fill those needs, we are free to create our Selves in our own image. We are no longer a slave to old, habitual, and many times self defeating images that no longer serve us.

When we respond to our own needs with a desire, the conscious mind draws upon related memories to help form the desire-thought that will be recreated by our subconscious mind as a condition in our outer lives. Using the example of the new boss, we begin to remember times we were in a position of authority. We recall a lecture we gave to a club, or an essay we had published, or the work we accomplished that earned us a raise. We remember images of others in authority positions who we admire: teachers, parents, political or social leaders. Using memory productively, we begin to imagine how we can draw upon our own successes and emulate those we admire to produce the desired respect and prestige in our lives now. As we imagine what if I looked this way, what if I spoke this way, what if I held this attitude, what if I made these suggestions, what if I offered to assist my boss or asked for more work or let it be known I am willing to work overtime, we begin to form our desire-thought. We create our Selves in our own image with full awareness of the expected outcome.

This causes the desire-thought to be impressed in the innermost level of the subconscious mind. Here the reflected image of our conscious creation acts as a seed idea finding a home in the receptive mind substance. Much like the reflected light image that is impressed upon camera film, the reflected image of your desire-thought begins to move through developmental stages. The seed of your desire-thought grows and matures in the inner levels of consciousness in your subconscious mind. Being transformed by energy acting upon the substance in your inner mind, the desire-thought experiences a period of incubation in the four elemental structures and eventually culminates in the physical manifestation of what you desire.

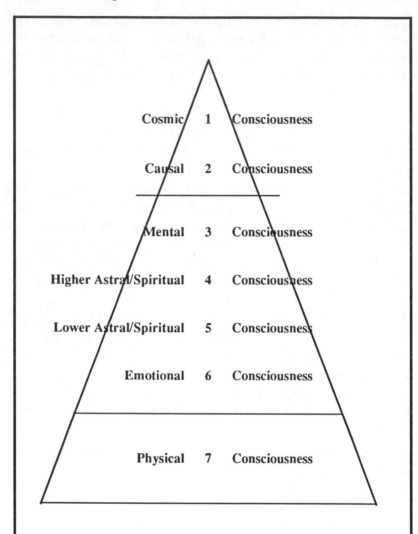

Cosmic 1 Consciousness

Causal 2 Consciousness

Mental 3 Consciousness

Higher Astral/Spiritual 4 Consciousness

Lower Astral/Spiritual 5 Consciousness

Emotional 6 Consciousness

Physical 7 Consciousness

Structure of the Inner Levels
of Consciousness
Two Dimensional Representation

The developmental stages of your desire-thought are determined by the qualities of the inner levels of the subconscious mind. Planted as a seed idea in the innermost expression of the subconscious mind, the mental level, your desire-thought is receptive to the energy and substance of this level of consciousness. When the desire-thought has received enough third level mind substance, it becomes aggressive pushing outward to the next outer level of the subconscious mind, the higher astral level, which is receptive to the growing seed idea. Here the desire-thought becomes receptive to the energy and substance of this level of consciousness, and this process is repeated until physical manifestation occurs. Because energy and substance are used in any visualizing endeavor, a means of replenishing the used energy and rejuvenating the substance is needed for life to continue. This recycling is the duty of the chakra system. Knowing how to replenish energy is a prerequisite for wielding Kundalini energy and knowledge of the inner levels of consciousness accelerates our ability to repeatedly draw upon her.

The first step for the awakened consciousness is to take care in the quality of the desire-thoughts created. For the novice, once your desire-thought is given to your subconscious mind, your conscious mind need only cooperate with the inner mind for development to occur. If you become impatient, the desire will manifest incompletely just as a photo pulled from developing solution will be out of focus and over exposed. If you refuse to cooperate, denying your original desire, you will retard its manifestation just as a photo that is left in developing solution too long will deteriorate. With cooperation, you will find a replica of what you have imaged just as a perfect photo, manifesting in your life.

The more you use visualization with awareness, you will pave the way for Kundalini to become active in your life, for the more you create, the more opportunities you produce for expanding your consciousness to include the infinite. You begin to define your identity as a thinker reaching to emulate the qualities of the intelligence which brought you into being. Just as a child imitates his physical parents, the maturing thinker causes his mind to expand through deep contemplation worthy of a creator of the universe. In this way, Man emulates his Spiritual parent.

As visualization becomes a skill, your proficiency in its use will grow. So will your questions concerning the purpose for your creative power. As you develop confidence in your ability to manifest any desire, you will eventually tire of your "Midas touch" unless you realize a higher purpose in your creative endeavors. When your consciousness has sufficiently expanded to embrace your spiritual essence, visualization will become a means for maturing your creative intelligence. Spiritual maturity is a harbinger for the mastery of Kundalini.

In Mind First

Everything in our physical existence first began in the inner levels of consciousness. Guided by the Universal Law of Duality, the aggressive and receptive principles are called into action. When they cooperate and harmonize creation occurs. Through spontaneous awakenings of Kundalini man enters realms of thought and existence previously alien to his view of life. Only by experience in the inner realms of existence can man expect to reveal the true nature of his own creativity. Through acts of creation, he comes to know Self as a creator. This is the enlightenment we seek.

To this point we have examined man's creative ability from the outside working inward. To more fully understand the importance of Kundalini in the dawning of a new and expansive consciousness, let us explore creation from the beginning of our existence. Whether we explore creation philosophically or scientifically, we find the essence of creation is light. Spiritually light is the building block for consciousness because it represents awareness. Scientifically light, known as the photon, is the building block for all physical forms.

Since the universe is filled with order and structure, there are no accidents or coincidences. From the first creation of light, evolution begins as a result of the needs and desires of an individual thinker. We have already examined how needs become apparent to the conscious mind, thus stimulating the visualization process. The same principles hold true throughout every stage of creation for this is the inherent and innate urge of the thinker - to be like his Creator through progressive acts of creation.

Throughout creation we find the expression of duality in the nature of balance and imbalance. Once balance is achieved another imbalance will become apparent because the inner urge of the thinker is to evolve and mature. Man's existence is dual in nature. The building blocks of life, scientifically termed DNA, are dual in nature being both spiritual and physical. DNA gives creative maturity structure and order serving as a place of origin for further development. Physically this is evidenced by a child growing in its mother's womb. The embryo will mature into a fetus then into a child. As this vehicle is built it grows through all physical DNA stages previously established in what we will call root races. These evolutionary developmental stages are so named because *root* denotes a point of origin and *race* describes a particular structure available for the consciousness to express through and gain experience.

In order for light to evolve the need became apparent to have a form through which first experience could be gained. This need birthed desire or an "I want" consciousness present in the spiritual DNA of every part of creation. "I want" finds its physical expression in the photon.

Once the thinker gains experience through this form, becoming familiar with its quality and expression, another need becomes apparent. This need is for mobility. The "I want" consciousness birthed in the first root continues and we find the desire for motion becomes a part of the spiritual DNA. The physical form evolves in response to this desire as atoms become attractive forces combining to form gases which is the first root race.

As the thinker gains experience through the form of gases, the need for stability arises. The desire to withstand force without alteration of position is found through the creation of minerals, the second root race.

Once the thinker gains experience through the form of minerals, the need for feeling arises. The desire to relate and respond to other parts of creation produces an "I want" for emotion. This is found in plant life, the third root race. In plant life we find the development of the nervous system, but it lacks mobility for there is no choice of what response will be given to external stimuli. The plant merely reacts to its environment.

Having gained experience through this form, the need for freedom of motion again arises. The desire to discriminate births the instinct apparent in the fourth root race, animals. Here we find the beginning of the formation of the brain and again the lack of choice in the vehicle to be used for experiencing.

Once the thinker gains experience through the form of animals, the need for volition arises. This need births the desire for reasoning which is characteristic of animal man, the fifth root race. Now we find the further development of the brain that will house memory and provide the mechanical tools necessary for imagination to be used by the thinker. This combined with the juxtapositioning of the thumb and fingers physically sets animal man apart from all other animals and frees the thinker to greatly accelerate his evolutionary process. Volition also gives man the ability to become cognizant of Kundalini energy and direct its use toward evolutionary progression. This is the stage of evolution we currently experience.

As reasoning becomes a part of the thinker, the need for the direct experience of truth becomes apparent. The desire for intuition forms in man's consciousness and the vehicle of Spiritual man is born as the sixth root race. As intuition is respected and embraced man integrates his consciousness and opens his awareness to the continuity of existence and his connectedness with the universe. He has learned to use Kundalini energy to reach the transcendental states of awareness and is no longer bound to the earth plane.

Having evolved through these root races, the need to create arises birthing a desire to be a creator compatible to the Spiritual Parent which provided our origin of existence. Thus Godman is the anticipated seventh root race.

The creative power known as the Kundalini is a spiritual energy effective in the physical. It is only with the development of the individual soul during the fifth root race that man achieves the elevated consciousness required to use the Kundalini energy. Earlier root races enjoy this flow of creative energy which enables physical procreation to occur, but they lack the necessary experience and understanding to harness her spiritual powers. By the time reasoning is developed, the thinker can realize his individual ability to guide his evolutionary development through the choices he makes. The acceptance of the responsibility for volition elevates man's awareness to consider his purpose for existence and awaken to his need for spiritual progression. This prepares his consciousness for the conscious use of the Kundalini energy.

One who has sufficiently expanded his consciousness, realizes the duality of his existence. He knows there are two worlds of existence: the physical world experienced through the five physical senses and the spiritual world experienced through mental attention and perception. This heightens his ability to function in more levels of consciousness opening his awareness of time as a measurement of progression. He realizes time is dual in nature. He knows horizontal time is measured by his experiences and vertical time is measured by his understanding of those experiences. The first is time registered in the brain, the latter is time registered in the soul. The first is the time required to live a full lifetime in the physical plane, the latter is the time invested in making Universal Truth a permanent part of the Self.

A metaphysician understands the origin of what can be perceived with the five physical senses of sight, sound, taste, touch, and smell. With the Greek word *meta* meaning "after" and *physikos* meaning "nature", metaphysics can be described as the exploration and knowledge of the Universal Laws which govern our existence. This knowledge frees man's consciousness to learn from, abide with, and make use of all of creation. It is interesting to note that the word "physics" is also akin to the Greek *phyo* meaning "to bring forth", and *phyo* has its origin in the Sanskrit *bhu* meaning "to be". Thus, to be a metaphysician means bringing awareness of the universe to Self by becoming a creator in your own right. In the world's Holy scriptures, man's origin is described as being divine, as being from a Creator, and his purpose for existing is to be like the Creator which brought him into existence. For millenniums, the Creator's offspring has evolved in consciousness to reach the point of awareness embodied as Reasoning Man. The acceleration of Reasoning Man's evolution, your evolution, is the reason to cause the Kundalini to rise.

The world's spiritual literature is metaphorical stories conveying the spiritual potential of man. These parables, myths, and legends put us in touch with our spiritual life. The goal of man's early existence as Reasoning Man was to live in constant awareness of Spiritual principles. Some of this has been lost in the material creations and advancements of recent centuries. The awakening of Kundalini beckons, indeed commands, that man rekindle his desire for Spiritual knowledge, experience and understanding. Since scientific exploration of Kundalini is deficit in the present time, a study of spiritual literature stimulates the mind toward acceptance and comprehension of experiences born from the aroused Kundalini.

The account of the man, the woman, and the serpent in the Garden of Eden is a Hebrew myth borrowed from an earlier Babylonian legend revealing the nature of consciousness. To those who think in linear, physical ways, this passage appears to be an account of what is commonly called the "fall of man" complete with malevolent evil, damning temptation, blame and regret. For those who think physically, this story becomes a deceptive illusion to explain the difficulties in their lives offering a scapegoat as the cause of man's misery. For those willing to remove the shackles of limitation bred by complacent yielding to ignorance, what has been kept secret for centuries can become known.

When we examine this Biblical passage with keen discernment and open-minded study, we can decipher the universal symbols used to reveal the relationships that compose man's inner consciousness and his urge to be like his Creator. In this way, we can learn about the structure of inner and outer consciousness for Reasoning Man. Let us examine this passage looking for truth that can be applied universally.

The story begins by describing the serpent as *"the most cunning of all the animals that the Lord God had made."* The Lord God implies a singular experience of creation. If we are to understand spiritual literature as revelatory of our inner condition, this would represent our true individuality, a recognition of existence that can be termed "I Am". I Am says I exist. It is a state of being at a point of origin where there is awareness of a Creator. Animals function from instinct or compulsion, so this would be an image indicating unconscious patterns of thinking. The serpent however is distinguished from all other forms of compulsive thinking because it is described as the most cunning. The word cunning comes from the Gothic *kunnan* meaning to know. Thus the serpent represents the desire for knowledge or wisdom. The serpent is an image used repeatedly in spiritual literature to describe the Kundalini energy.

In the story of creation, man is created in the image and after the likeness of his Creator. This indicates the birth of an intelligence, aggressive or male in quality, which is created from thought and contains similar attributes to its Creator. Spiritually we are our Father's son. As the description continues the intelligence becomes dual adding the quality of receptivity required for the intelligence *"to be like"* his maker. The Lord God creates a suitable partner for the man by removing one of his ribs and forming a woman. This illustrates the further structuring of consciousness we have described as the subconscious mind *(man)* and the conscious mind *(wo-man)*.

The serpent asks the woman, *"Did God really tell you not to eat from any of the trees of the garden?"* This interchange between the serpent and the woman represents the stimulation of the desire for knowledge and wisdom in the conscious mind. The desire is to receive knowledge *(eat)* through the use of the centers in the brain *(trees of the garden)*. The woman in the story responds to the serpent saying," *We may eat of the fruit of the trees in the garden; it is only about the fruit of the tree in the middle of the garden that God said, 'You shall not eat it or even touch it, lest you die.'"* She, the conscious mind, is assessing what has been used to this time for learning. The brain has been used in every way except to change *(die)* consciousness. Remember it is with the need for volition that animal man, the fifth root race, is produced. Until this occurs, learning is instinctual rather than the result of aware choice. From the impetus toward reasoning - the cunning of the serpent - the conscious mind begins to reach.

The serpent replies to the woman: *"You certainly will not die! No, God knows well that the moment you eat of it your eyes will be opened and you will be like gods who know what is good and what is bad."* By using the imagery of the serpent, this story describes the motivating force in mind that propels discovery. By stimulating the conscious mind to use information already gathered, the serpent becomes the expression of our individual desire to grow. We experience this as ego. The ego expresses itself through the desire for perception *(eyes will be opened)* and for the creativity *(be like gods)* that is produced by reasoning *(know what is good and what is bad)*. Because the ego's function is to motivate the conscious mind into action, there is no recognition of the changes this knowledge will bring. This becomes the pattern for the relationship between the conscious mind and the conscious expression of ego.

The story continues describing how the woman eats of the fruit of the tree and gives some to her husband. Their eyes are opened and they realize they are naked. They sew fig leaves to make loincloths. The conscious mind responds to the ego's motivation taking in knowledge from experiences. As it is assimilated, the knowledge is given to the subconscious mind *(man)* bringing the recognition of what has been caused *(eyes of both were opened)*. The result of this knowledge is a realization of the lack of experience *(naked)* and the need to produce experiences *(loincloths)*.

The man and woman hide when the Lord God appears in the Garden. The time of innocence is past and responsibility for learning has been set into motion. Once awareness of what has occurred reaches the I Am, there is a recognition that the means of learning will now need to change in response to the conscious mind's newly developed ability to reason.

In the following verses from the book of *Genesis*, we find the symbolic initiation of three significant parts of what is now Reasoning Man's identity. We find each has a specific duty and purpose relative to the others. Each also has a unique expression of what will often be referred to in this writing as the inner urge to evolve. These changes are described in the following verses:

> *Then the Lord God said to the serpent:*
> *"Because you have done this, you shall be banned from all the animals and from all the wild creatures; On your belly shall you crawl, and dirt shall you eat all the days of your life.*
> *I will put enmity between you and the woman, and between your offspring and hers;*
> *He will strike at your head while you strike at his heel."*

As you have by now noticed, it is the true individuality, the I Am, that guides the evolutionary development of the thinker. Here we find the seat of the desire to be like, to mature as a creator. Thus the I Am delineates the means by which maturity can occur. The expression of the ego in the physical is given purpose and direction. It will be separate from the brain pathways of compulsive thinking *(banned from all animals...)*, yet find its means of performing its duty to motivate from what has been stored as memory in the substance of the brain *(dirt shall you eat...)*. Man's conscious sense of identity will no longer be based upon instinct, rather it will be the result of constant stimulation between the conscious ego and the conscious mind *(enmity between you and the woman)*. The purpose of the ego will be to constantly present the conscious mind with motivation to form the identity through expanding old ideas of Self into new ideas of Self *(between your offspring and hers)*. It will bring constant stimulation of the desire "to be like" to the conscious mind *(he will strike at your head...)* until full maturity of the reasoning ability is achieved. It is interesting to note that the Oriental symbol for everlasting life is the serpent with its head in its mouth, a suitable representation of the inner urge of the conscious ego to mature for full realization of the inner Ego, the I Am.

> *To the woman he said:*
> *"I will intensify the pangs of your childbearing;*
> *in pain shall you bring forth children. Yet your*
> *urge shall be for your husband, and he shall be*
> *your master."*

The relationship of the conscious ego to the conscious mind having been established, the I Am now determines the duty and purpose of the conscious mind. The power of the conscious mind is the ability to reason. Established as the discriminatory power to identify what is productive and what is nonproductive for growth as symbolized by the woman eating of the tree of knowledge, this conscious mind is from this time forward responsible for the use of this power. Through reasoning, the conscious mind's duty is to produce new forms of thinking and new ways of life *(bring forth children)* to further evolution. These new ideas will be conceived as a result of what is needed for maturity of Self to occur. When there is not awareness of what is lacking in Self or when there is a lack of understanding of how to create *(intensify the pangs of your childbearing)*, there will still be the constant stimulation for the conscious mind to use reasoning from the ego. As reasoning produces experiences for the conscious mind, the opportunity for understanding is made available thus giving the conscious mind its purpose. The understandings gained are given to the subconscious mind to be stored in the permanent memory of the soul *(your urge shall be for your husband)*. In this way, these understood experiences become a permanent part of the identity *(he shall be your master)*. The inner urge of the conscious mind is to experience physical life for the purpose of producing the understandings necessary to become a creator.

> *To the man he said:*
> *"Because you listened to your wife and ate from the tree of which I had forbidden you to eat, Cursed be the ground because of you! In toil shall you eat its yield all the days of your life. Thorns and thistles shall it bring forth to you, as you eat of the plants of the field. By the sweat of your face shall you get bread to eat, until you return to the ground, from which you were taken; For you are dirt, and to dirt you shall return."*

The duty of the subconscious mind is to receive the new ideas created by the conscious mind *(because you listened to your wife)*. Its function will be to reproduce any desire *(thorns and thistles)* the conscious mind produces through the process of manifestation *(in toil shall you eat its yield...)*. The subconscious mind will also maintain the life force systems *(as you eat of the plants of the field)* necessary for the conscious mind to be able to continue experiencing. By fulfilling its duty, the subconscious mind's purpose of storing the understood experiences necessary for maturity can be fulfilled *(by the sweat of your face shall you get bread to eat)*. The inner urge of the subconscious mind will be the fulfillment of knowing how to form mind substance *(return to the ground, from which you are taken)*. And the subconscious mind will continue to exist as part of the identity of man until this has been completed *(For you are dirt, and to dirt you shall return)*.

The story ends with the man naming his wife Eve because she is to become *"the mother of all the living"*. A new relationship of the subconscious mind and the conscious mind is now established. The conscious mind, through its ability to create *(mother of all the living)*, will now dictate the quality and rate of learning for the whole Self. When the conscious mind reaches to develop its creative ability, discovery occurs. The more expansive the conscious thinking, the more far-reaching are the effects of its creations. The more we exercise a willingness to birth new ideas, the more we accelerate our own and others evolution.

We know good from evil, right from wrong, what will produce in harmony with Universal Law and what will not. This is the message in eating from the tree of good and evil. Far from being an act of unworthiness or reason for disgrace, the activity described in the Garden of Eden reveals the inner spiritual connections that give man the ability to reason and the power of creative discovery.

The Garden of Eden represents a place of unity, a place where man and woman dwell in the presence of God. It symbolizes the place of origin and the place of destination in man's spiritual journey for it is also where the tree of life exists. The tree of life gives knowledge of immortality. The real challenge of Kundalini begins with the tree of life. When she is awakened we come to know enlightenment as reflected in the statement "I and the Father are One." We transcend the boundaries of mortal thinking and enter into the omnipresence of continual existence.

When Yahweh, or the Lord God, expels the man and woman from the Garden he places at its entrance two cherubim and a flaming sword. This represents the challenge of raising the Kundalini to produce revelation in consciousness. Man must expand his consciousness of Spirit *(cherubim)* to become free from the earth plane by resolving his karmic indebtedness *(flaming sword)*. Only then will he gain transcendental knowledge of his immortality.

This imagery is also seen in Buddhist teachings. At the entrance of Buddhist shrines sits the Buddha under the tree of immortal life. On each side of him are two guardians or cherubim, one with its mouth open and one with its mouth closed representing the pairs of opposites. When you approach, if you are unprepared, these two will threaten you, denying you entrance into the shrine. Only your own unresolved fears and desires can keep you from entering your own temple and experiencing your immortality. Your Spirit is ever-present, awaiting the moment when you will transcend limitation and enter into the enlightened state of being described by all the great masters of our history.

The Triad of Creative Intelligence

Each of us has moments in our lives when we question the cause of our existence. Usually, this soul-searching is in response to a physical stimulus and accompanied by extreme emotional reactions. It is as if life inherently holds experiences which momentarily rouse our sleeping consciousness into a state of Self awareness and discovery.

Most come to the point of asking "why" when confronted with their own mortality. The death of a peer, a life-threatening disease, or witnessing physical abuse via live television can serve as the stimulus. It is what and how you think about these life events that will promote Self awareness or perpetuate ignorance. When Self awareness is your answer, you recognize opportunities for realizing the continuity of your existence as Spirit. Just as emotions of sorrow, anxiety, and confusion can serve to expand consciousness so can more positive emotions of joy, excitement, and anticipation. A wedding, the birth of a child, or a graduation or promotion all serve as a physical stimulus providing an incentive for us to recognize our reason to exist. No matter what conditions are manifested in our life, the seed idea for our growth as a creator remains. Midst the temporal conditions of our physical life, that seed is a constant.

Beyond your ability to manifest conditions in your life, is your potential to understand the nature of creativity from a creator's viewpoint. Through knowing the inner components of creation, Self awareness is heightened because you come face to face with your Spiritual parentage. To know Self beyond the limitations of the physical, is to set the mind free to contemplate the powers of the universe. There are forces active in our universe which affect and give order to existence. These forces can be termed Universal Laws and Principles for they are neutral in action, operating at any time, at any place, upon any one in our realm of existence.

The pursuit of knowledge of these Universal Laws has been the objective of Reasoning Man for thousands of years. The world's myths and legends have evolved as a way to describe the mysteries of the universe and man's relationship to the source of his being. These metaphorical and allegorical stories at first were passed down from generation to generation through the art of story-telling. Each time the story was told, the one describing the imagery was changed. This continues to be true, for with direct experience of mind-expanding literature consciousness finds food for thought.

In more recent years, many of the tales have been recorded and become widely published as the Holy scriptures of the world. The fact that they are described as holy can be seen as reference to their content revolving around universal and godly matters. Perhaps even more appropriate the word implies a whole concept or idea which transcends all limitation. As we move further in our exploration of Kundalini, we will refer often to these texts, myths, and legends for the universal insights they reveal.

The forces which order our universe can be found in most Holy scriptures. For instance, they are described in the ten commandments of the Bible, the Eight Fold Path of Buddha, or the tenets of the Tao Te Ching. In more recent times, science has become acquainted with the workings of these laws through the observation of their physical expression, such as the Law of Gravity. Current experimentation in quantum physics leads scientists to explore metaphysical realms of existence and to consider the realities beyond the physical senses.

Wherever man may be in his search for truth in understanding the nature of Self and his universe, it remains universally true that man is a thinker and his essence is spirit. Esoterically, there are three principles guiding spirit. In Hindu writings these are termed Creative Intelligence, Akasha, and Prana. Becoming familiar with the universal nature of these principles and with their influence in your own movement of thinking aids you in understanding and using the Kundalini energy available to you. Here we also find the origin and evolution of man's inherent ability to create.

These three appear through spiritual literature in the triune gods. They are represented in Celtic myths as Odin, the father, Frea his wife and the universal mother, and Thor, their son or the mediator. In the Christian tradition they are the Father, Son, and Holy Spirit. In Hindu they are known as Brahma, Shiva, and Vishnu. These can be described as faith or true wisdom, hope or the strength insuring achievement, and charity or the service which makes united effort possible.

The first of this triad, Creative Intelligence, finds its origin as the spark of life from its Creator. Scientifically, we find this to be described as a building block, the photon, existing in all of creation. A photon is an electromagnetic wave of light present in all atomic structures. In Holy scriptures, the initial creation of the Creator is described as Light, indicating awareness. Where there is awareness, there is identity. Identity feeds the awareness of existence and in its movement we find volition. This produces the individuality known as the *I Am* in man.

In each individual, there exists a deeper level of awareness beyond the subconscious and conscious minds. This superconscious mind is closest to the true individuality of Self. Often symbolized in world mythologies as the mother and the father, the superconscious mind has a duty and purpose to fulfill. The duty of the superconscious mind is to supply energy to the outer parts of mind for their continued existence. This constant outpouring of energy insures that learning can transpire for the purpose of maturing the whole Self.

Creative Intelligence in Reasoning Man comes to life as the inner urge to be like his Creator. Just as a growing child will imitate his parents in word and action, so man imitates his Spiritual parent. Man's inner urge is fueled by his curiosity and desire for discovery. For thousands of years this manifested in explorations of "the new world". Now it continues in explorations of outer space. Whether five thousand years ago or today, the conscious mind of man responds to the inner urge to be like his maker through the use of imagination and will. With imagination, we can perceive the unknown factors of creation. Our ability to make these factors known is an act of will.

When we become skillful reasoners, the direct grasp of truth described as knowing produces intuition. Each time you visualize on purpose and with purpose you cause a harmonization of your conscious and subconscious minds. By expanding conscious awareness to parts of Self existing beyond the physical - the body and brain, the conscious mind and ego - the workings of the subconscious mind become familiar. As a storehouse for understandings, the inner levels of existence afford the thinker the wisdom gained through experience extending far beyond his present physical identity. Through repeated visualization, inner rapport develops which can be drawn upon unconsciously during dream states or consciously during meditation. This opens awareness to intuitive abilities such as clairvoyance, clairaudience, psychometry, and telepathy. Mastery of intuition is a further use of Creative Intelligence, and it is the next stage in man's evolution.

The principle of Akasha guides the substance of man's existence. Akasha is the inner substance needed for the creation of thought. Depending upon the unique forms constructed, the thinker owes his continuing existence as an individual, separate from other forms of creation, to this principle. The forms created in akasha distinguish individuality whether these are distinct thought forms or the myriad arrangements of atomic elements.

This is easy to comprehend when we consider the final manifestation of akasha: physical matter. Your physical body is constructed of akasha commonly described as cells. Each cell of your body is whole and complete. Each cell contains the essence of physical life, the DNA code which is the manifestation of the blueprint for your physical existence. From this blueprint a complete and whole physical body can be produced, a clone of your physical existence. Fascinating in its existence, the cell is the reflection of the inner urge "to be like" found in the innermost part of the thinker.

Just as the cell is a manifestation in akasha of the purpose for your existence, it also displays remarkable manifestations of mental abilities in its function and duty. There are six characteristics in the functioning of the cell. These are irritability, contractility, metabolism, reproduction, conductivity, and adaptability. The mind's receptivity to stimulus is manifested in irritability or the cell's ability to react to a stimulus. The mind's aggressiveness is manifested in contractility or the ability to move. The mind's ability to think and comprehend manifests in the cell's metabolism. The mind's ability to recreate manifests in the cell's ability for reproduction. The mind's ability to coordinate and harmonize aggressive and receptive qualities shows in the cell's ability to carry a positive or negative charge. The mind's ability to use a vehicle for experiencing manifests in the cell's ability to adjust to and use the environment. Each of these are manifestations of Universal Laws and Principles which are first evidenced in consciousness. This is the reason your body will reflect the attitudes you hold in mind creating either health or disease.

Your physical body occupies a specific space effectively expressing your chosen identity as a male or female, as a child or as an adult. We even use substance to aid us in defining who we are by alterations in the way we look according to our Self image and our desire for status or recognition in relationship with others. Akasha also affirms our individuality by separating us from other forms of substance such as the chair you are sitting on, the building you are in, or the other person in the room.

Anyone practicing creation knows the need for substance. For instance, an artist must have mediums for the mental creations he envisions to be given physical life. If he is a sculptor, he will use substance such as clay to shape and mold a representation of the image he holds in his mind. Once the imaged form desired is reproduced in physical form, his creation can be shared with others. The artist has effectively molded substance so others can experience through their senses his vision.

The existence of substance and our ability to manipulate the form it takes, shows the relationship between the principles of Akasha and Creative Intelligence. This frees us to both give and receive experience necessary for our evolution, and when this occurs the third principle, Prana, is called into action. Prana is a Sanskrit word meaning *absolute energy*. The mental energy the artist uses to envision his masterpiece finds its intelligent direction in the artist's will. Through causing movement in thought, he can arrange memory images and create new thought forms in the akasha present in the inner levels of his consciousness. By willing his body and hands to be energized, he can manipulate and change the shape of the clay to match his desired image. Even the clay, his substance of choice, owes its flexibility and moldability to the principle of prana.

The subtle inner workings of the artist's mind illustrate the individual principles of creation and their interdependent relationship which enables all of us to experience the manifest likeness of our thoughts. One of these inner workings necessary for this to occur is described as the chakra system.

The word *chakra* is Sanskrit meaning circle or wheel. In most esoteric literature, chakras are described in relationship to energy only, probably because their main function is to transform energy. Yet, these wheels of life draw upon all of the principles of creation. Their effectiveness as energy transformers depends upon the kinds of thoughts we create and the quality of the inner substance being molded. In this way, each chakra responds to particular types of vibratory thought similar to how a radio receiver responds to a specific frequency signal. Once the soul incarns, the chakra frequencies are set into motion as a result of evolutionary development. As conscious thinking develops, each chakra directs the transference of energy associated with specific vibrations of thought. This transference of energy can perform whatever functions are necessary to maintain life.

Chakras are also responsive to the energy required by substance to sustain a form; this substance being the inner and outer body of man. Thus when any body is in an energy deficit condition, the corresponding chakra will endeavor to cause balance in that area by resupplying it with energy. You may have experienced this replenishing as spontaneous bursts of energy or as warm currents running through your body without knowing their origin. This will occur when your attention is directed toward Self mentally and emotionally, most often as a result of a creative endeavor. If the energy supply remains deficit in an area over a period of time, the form will begin to break down. In the body this state is referred to as disease which is the result of prolonged negative thinking.

Chakra functions are necessary to sustain life enabling the thinker's existence for further creation and growth. The functions of returning energy in this way are dictated by what can be termed spiritual DNA. Just as the evolutionary development of man's physical body can be studied in the genetic code of its DNA, man's evolutionary development as Reasoning Man can be studied by examining the nature and structure of his spirituality. As the superconscious mind energizes the subconscious mind which in turn energizes the conscious mind, energy is available for conscious reasoning and creativity. The chakras exist to enable this energy to be recycled and used again. By understanding the major chakras, you will gain insight into the relationship they have with the directed use of creative energy we call the Kundalini. You will also become familiar with ways you can develop your consciousness in preparation for using Kundalini.

There are ten major chakras functioning in man. For full consciousness to be achieved, all must be used with conscious awareness by the thinker. Each chakra functions as a vortex, continually in motion, drawing cosmic energy into the inner levels of consciousness. The action can be likened to a vortex of

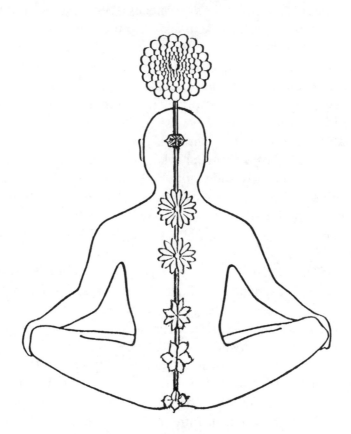

The Lotuses
of the Seven Chakra System

water swirling down a drain or substance passing through a funnel. Centripetal force draws the energy inward for transformation in preparation for reuse. When the Kundalini is awakened, this natural movement of the chakras is altered, drawing energy out of the inner levels of consciousness by centrifugal force for immediate manifestation of the desired thought. The Kundalini is the most powerful spiritual energy available to man. Inner knowledge and spiritual practices will prepare you for her use.

In esoteric literature, the chakras are often symbolized by the unfolding petals of the lotus. The lotus is sacred in India. Growing from mud, the lotus symbolizes the path of development from primitive and limited awareness to fully blossoming and expansive consciousness. Like the lotus, chakras have petals, and like a flower, they vary in size, color, and brilliance. The energy flow through each chakra forms a particular configuration or pattern. As the configuration blossoms, vibrations begin to form shaping the size, variation in color, speed of rotation, and rhythm of each individual chakra. Each chakra's interconnection with other centers produces the quality and character of the whole Self. The degree of function of each chakra will reflect the strength of the connection with the developed consciousness in the individual.

Seven of the major centers are fields of physiological, electromagnetic, mental, and spiritual energy. In the inner planes of existence, chakras are points of intersection between these planes. Their existence in the vehicle for the subconscious mind, the soul, can be perceived with the sixth sense. They find their final expression in the physical body in conjunction with the seven ductless glands and in the five lower chakras with the nerve plexuses of the autonomic nervous system.

When the flow of energy being returned by any chakra is interrupted, that chakra is often described as being "blocked" which actually indicates a decrease in energy being recycled. This will occur when Creative Intelligence is being misused as in times of fear, ignorance, or the stress of negative thinking. These conditions vary widely in the life of each individual.

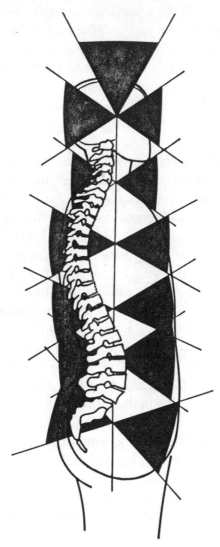

The Seven Major Chakra Centers
and Their Physiological Fields

Indications of which chakras are blocked can be realized by noting parts of the physical body that are restricted or signalling pain. Physical symptoms are indications that the chakra associated with the area is not processing all of the energy flowing through it. For instance, headaches can result when the sixth chakra, the brow, energy is restricted. Tightness in the throat, neck, and shoulders can result from improper function of the fifth chakra, the throat. When a chakra remains blocked for an extended period of time, disease will manifest in the body. For instance, when the fourth chakra, the heart, is blocked palpitations in the heart will result. If allowed to continue over a period of time, heart disease will eventually manifest.

Most people are absorbed by their animal nature and physical bodies. Being attached to people, places, and things in the physical, they live predominantly in the thinking governing the three lower chakras. These people limit their awareness of who they are lacking understanding of their purpose for existence as a thinker. They are tied to the wheel of death and rebirth, insuring the need for future incarnations until they achieve states of enlightened consciousness. When an individual uses creativity in his physical life he will draw primarily on the energies of the five lower chakras. Those who exhibit genius are drawing on all chakra energies with or without awareness and often experience the spontaneous awakening of Kundalini energies.

As you become familiar with the purpose and function of the major chakras, you will also become acquainted with specific creative processes that will influence their functioning. By directing creativity, you call upon your Kundalini energy to cause a change in your awareness elevating your state of consciousness. This change causes your use of energy to be complete. When allowed to function properly, the chakras will return the energy you have used in visualization to the inner levels of your consciousness. This strengthens your mind and body preparing them for the onset of Kundalini activity. Through investment of time in study and application of spiritual disciplines you can expect to gain awareness whereby you can consciously direct the power of the creative energies present in us all.

The Seven Major Chakras
and their Physical Correspondence to the Body

All chakra centers exist beyond the physical with their actions affecting the energies in the physical body. As mental energy is used and recycled, its expression can be noted in the physical plane of existence. Before we delve into the causal principles of each chakra, let us explore how the movement of energy makes itself known in the workings of the body.

In relationship to the physical body, the chakras are located where two major etheric energy currents, known as the *ida* and the *pingala* in Eastern philosophies, crisscross over a major flow of energy in the center of the spinal column. This major flow is known as *sushumna*. The light of consciousness travels through the sushumna feeding and drawing upon the chakra centers for the ultimate purpose of enlightenment. This is the pathway of the Kundalini when it is rising up the spine to the brain.

The ida energy current rules the left side of the body finding its physical expression in the parasympathetic nervous system. Esoterically, ida is described as the moon representing the receptive principle of creative energy. The pingala energy current rules the right side of the body finding its expression in the sympathetic nervous system. Esoterically, pingala is de-

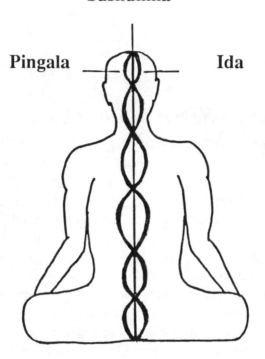

Sushumna

Pingala **Ida**

Major Energy Currents
(back view of spinal column)

scribed as the sun representing the aggressive principle of creative energy. Together, these two energy flows form what is known as the autonomic nervous system in the physical body.

For most people, cardiac muscle and smooth muscle function involuntarily and beyond conscious control. Smooth muscle is found in the organs of the digestive, respiratory, circulatory and urinogential systems, while cardiac muscle is found exclusively in the heart. These muscles are controlled by the autonomic nervous system composed of two seemingly opposing divisions. The sympathetic nerves leave the spinal cord in nerve chains before connecting the body organs where they stimulate muscle activity. When rapid action is required the sympathetic nervous system becomes dominant. For instance when the mind reacts in fear to perceived danger there is an increase in heart rate, respiration, blood pressure and sweat gland activity. In the parasympathetic nervous system, nerves pass from the spinal cord directly to the organs having the opposite effect of decreasing muscular activity. When the body is at rest, the parasympathetic system is dominant. This occurs usually during sleep when the heart rate is slower and respiration deeper and more regular. This rhythmic alternation in the activity of the sympathetic and parasympathetic nervous systems brings about peristalsis or natural motion required for proper organ function.

Medical scientists are beginning to realize what students of metaphysics have long practiced - the ability of mind to influence and direct matter. In the case of the autonomic nervous system, what is taken for granted as merely occurring without cause is appreciated and understood by one who regularly practices controlling the heartbeat and the breath. By consciously directing these subconscious functions, the thinker gains greater awareness and unites the inner and outer consciousness.

A common example of taking conscious control of involuntary autonomic functions is control of the bladder. When young, we learn to direct the function of the bladder. Physically, when the buildup of a large volume of urine occurs, the muscular wall is stretched signalling the parasympathetic system to contract

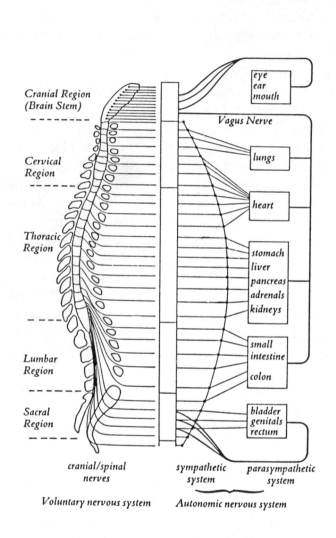

Cranial Region
(Brain Stem)

eye
ear
mouth

Vagus Nerve

Cervical
Region

lungs

heart

Thoracic
Region

stomach
liver
pancreas
adrenals
kidneys

small
intestine

colon

Lumbar
Region

Sacral
Region

bladder
genitals
rectum

cranial/spinal
nerves

sympathetic
system

parasympathetic
system

Voluntary nervous system   *Autonomic nervous system*

The Nervous Systems
of the Physical Body

the muscles of the bladder and relax the sphincter allowing release of the stored up urine. Our ability to control this autonomic function is learned as a part of social custom so we can choose the time we want this normal body process to occur. The same is true of the movement of the bowels. The primary motivation for taking control of these eliminatory functions is convenience. When man develops a purpose for controlling other autonomic functions, he will excel in his understanding of not only the physical body but more importantly of the advantages offered to his health and wholeness that such control can bring.   This type of initiative and the control it brings is a prerequisite for someone who desires to direct the flow of Kundalini energy at will.

The sushumna energy corresponds to the central nervous system consisting of the brain and spinal cord. This intricate channel of communication is also dual in nature. Afferent or sensory nerves convey incoming messages from sensory receptors and efferent or motor nerves carry outgoing messages to effector structures such as the voluntary muscles of the limbs. Sensory and motor nerves leave the spinal cord separately between the vertebrae but then unite to form thirty-one pairs of spinal nerves in which there are both sensory and motor nerve fibers. Leaving the brain directly are twelve pairs of cranial nerves. There are more than ten thousand million nerve units in the brain, but even these account for only one-tenth of the brain cells. It is the central nervous system which affords the intelligence that is you, the necessary "equipment" to gain experience in the physical level of consciousness.

Before the energy is manifested in the body as the central nervous system and autonomic nervous system, the finer, more subtle pranic energies emanate as the life force in man. As the energy currents of the ida and pingala move, they cross seven times, merging with the sushumna energy enabling integration and unification of the three energy flows. This unification allows creation to occur through the uniting of the aggressive and receptive principles with the lines of consciousness which govern creative activity.   Where these three energy fields meet in the spinal column, a chakra center is produced.

The seven centers represent intense fields of physiological, electromagnetic, mental, and spiritual energy. Physical organs, glands, and nerve plexuses are activated by subtle pulsations of energy at each center. The various functions and special forms of energy whirling through each center define the spiritual and physical qualities characteristic of each chakra. Just as iron filings form specific patterns reflecting the electromagnetic field of a nearby magnet, the energy flowing through the energy transformers also form particular patterns according to the energy field of the transformer. When perceived with the inner mind, each chakra can be distinguished according to its vibratory pattern. These will be reflected in the quality of thinking produced or used by the individual and will ultimately become physically manifested in the organs and body structure.

Though not physical, the chakras are positioned along the spinal column of the physical body. They closely correspond to the locations of the major nerve plexuses and endocrine glands. The human body works efficiently only when the equilibrium within each organ, tissue, and cell is closely monitored and controlled. Activity, growth and repair of tissues must be maintained as well as the supply of fuels and the removal of waste material.

These controls are achieved by two systems. The first is the network of nerve fibers which carry messages between the brain and the rest of the body. The second is the endocrine system. The word endocrine comes from the Greek words *endon* meaning within and *krinen* meaning to separate. This system is comprised of seven ductless glands which maintain the internal balance of the body. Each responds to a specific quality of inner thinking which governs a particular chakra. As a part of the physical body, the endocrine glands serve as a manifestation of the separateness of the thinker within from the outer vehicle he is using.

Endocrine glands release their chemical products or hormones directly into the bloodstream. These hormones are slower in action than nerve impulses, with the exception of the two hormones produced by the adrenal gland which act quickly and for a short time. Hormones travel through the bloodstream to every cell in the body. The membrane of each cell has receptors to one or more hormones, and the binding of a hormone to its specific cell receptor initiates particular changes in the internal metabolism of this "target" cell. In this way endocrine glands help control the internal environment and composition of each cell and organ in the physical body. When disease or imbalance is found in a gland of the physical body, you will find dis-ease or imbalance in the functioning of its corresponding chakra center not as a result of physical disease but as a causal agent.

Physically, the first chakra's energy influences the base of the spine and is related to the coccygeal spinal plexus and perineum or large bowel. The largest peripheral nerve in the body, the sciatic nerve, is also under the Root chakra's domain. The sciatic nerve is the root of the nervous system energy going to the feet and legs.

The chakra also influences the genitals and sacral plexus. In the gonads we find the polarization of male and female. Producing hormones for masculinizing and feminizing of the body, the reproductive organs perform specialized functions for the reproduction of the physical body. Sex hormones are responsible, along with genetic constitution, for the determination and maintenance of primary and secondary sexual differentiation. In a female body, ovaries produce ova, in the male body the testes produce spermatazoa. Both are germ cells for the perpetuation of the species. Another part of reproductive function is to produce hormones to maintain secondary sex characteristics, inducing reproductive cycles in the female and producing sperm in the male.

Each cell contains a genetic code physically governing its structure. There are 46 chromosomes, 23 sets of pairs or strands of DNA in each spermatazoan and each ovum. The arrangement and patterning of nucleotides comprise ultra-long DNA molecules that provide a biochemical template from which elements of the body are constructed such as individual characteristics and basic cellular mechanisms and molecular

The pineal gland is an internal clock related to reproduction and function of the entire endocrine system.

The hypothalamus controls pituitary secretions, body temperature, also hunger, thirst and sex drives.

The pituitary gland controls bone growth and regulates activity in other endocrine glands.

The thyroid gland controls the rate of fuel use in the body and body development.

The thymus controls the production of a type of infection-fighting white blood cell.

Adrenal glands control salt and water balance in the body and help prepare the body for emergencies.

The pancreas controls the level of sugar in the blood.

Ovaries in females control sexual development and the production of eggs.

Testes in males control sexual development and the production of sperm.

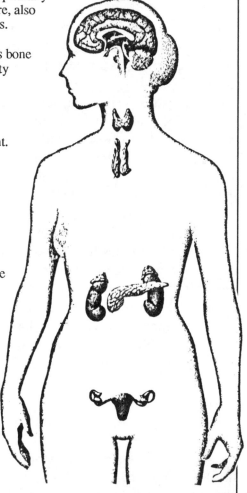

The Endocrine System

interactions. One pair of DNA holds the biochemical key to sexual polarity in what are termed sex chromosomes x(F) and y (M).

The second chakra's energy influences the adrenal (suprarenal) glands which are situated on top of kidneys. The adrenal cortex synthesizes forty different steroid substances for metabolism of the body. It is modulated by endocrine linkage to the anterior pituitary gland and the hypothalamus.

There are three primary steriods produced by the adrenal glands. *Aldosterone* which causes retention of sodium by stimulating reabsorption of sodium in kidneys and increasing the excretion of potassium, *glucocorticoids* which respond to stress, stimulate formation of glucose in liver and mobilization of fat (these also cause decrease in protein synthesis so amino acids increase in blood), and *mineralcorticoids* which react to ACTH from the pituitary to increase glucose and amino acids in blood. The male sex hormone androgen is also produced here.

The adrenal medulla produces catecholamines include adrenalin (epinephrine) which is linked to the sympathetic nervous system. The cells are located in clumps where sympathetic preganglionic nerve flow terminates. In Chinese acupuncture studies, adrenaline is described as yang owing to its aggressive nature. Adrenaline prepares the body for action to flee or defend by communication through the nervous system. Adrenaline gives us endurance. It is often called the emergency hormone for its rapid deployment of energy when stressed.

The third chakra's energy influences the celiac plexus and pancreas. Located over the adrenal glands, the celiac or solar plexus has a direct connection with the digestive system including the pancreas, liver, and stomach each required for the proper digestion of food. Particularly affected by this chakra's energy is the pancreas. The pancreas is both exocrine and endocrine in function. The exocrine glands secrete enzymes through ducts into the gut regulating carbohydrate, fat, and protein metabolism. More directly related to the chakra function are the endocrine cells found in the Islets of Langerhans. Over 200,000 of these cells are responsible for hormonal secretions which regulate insulin and glucogen storage creating a ready supply of body fuels.

The fourth chakra's energy influences the cardiac plexus and the thymus gland. The thymus is the center of the body's protective, immunological network. Located underneath the rib cage and close to heart, the thymus derived from the embryonic epithelium and is currently thought to lose its importance with age. However, the hormones involved with maturation of T cell lymphocytes (lymphocytes and leuocytes produced especially in spleen and bone marrow) are produced in the thymus. It is responsible for establishing a population of lymphocytes for cell mediated immunity. T lymphocytes have the capability to destroy foreign cells, and when the body ages they will migrate from the thymus to the lymph nodes and spleen.

We have previously spoken of the cardiac plexus as a part of the autonomic nervous system. Each day we take 18,000 to 20,000 breaths and can only go minutes without air. During normal respiration, most people only breathe in a pint of air per breath although the lungs will hold two pints of air. The breath is so important to the function of the physical body that a whole system of yoga, pranayama, is built on understanding and controlling its movement. To such a practitioner, breath means divine consciousness.

The fifth chakra's energy influences the thyroid and parathyroid glands. These glands perform a management function as general metabolic controllers. The thyroid secretes a hormone controlling the levels of body calcium which maintains the skeleton. It controls metabolism or the speed with which the body transforms nutrients into energy. When the rate is slightly lower than normal the body will experience fatigue. When slightly above normal, the body will experience hypersensitivity or nervousness. When markedly increased, weight loss, nervousness, a sense of being warm, and emotional disturbances will arise. When the metabolic rate is markedly decreased, a slowing of bodily functions eventually resulting in death occurs.

The parathyroid working with the thyroid maintains the level of calcium in the blood. An adult's body contain about 2.2

pounds of calcium, 99 percent of it is in the bones, the remainder in the blood stream. Calcium is important not only for bones and teeth but also for nerve function, muscle contraction, blood clotting, and glandular secretion. When you don't get enough calcium in your diet, the body takes it from your bones which can cause them to fracture spontaneously. Too much calcium in the blood leads to kidney stones and weakened muscle tone. Too little calcium can cause twitching, spasms, convulsions and even death.

The sixth chakra's energy influences the pituitary gland located in the brain below the hypothalamus and attached by a stalk with neural portion and glandular portion. The neural portion of the pituitary stores and secretes hormones produced by the hypothalamus. The glandular portion produces its own hormones which are released when stimulated by hypothalamic releasing hormones. The pituitary gland is the link between the nervous system and the endocrine system functioning as a servant of the hypothalamus.

This master gland of the body weighs only 1/50 of an ounce and is 85% water, yet it orchestrates and conducts the entire endocrine system. The pituitary monitors the action of the other glands and their production of hormones. For this reason, the pituitary is known as the chemical "boss" of body. When activated by stress or physical shock, the pituitary's lengthy amino acids will release endorphins, the body's natural pain killers. Endorphin levels have been linked to the pleasure level and states of unconditional joy. Laughter triggers its release, as can music, extended vigorous exercise, and Zen-yogic meditations.

The pituitary is composed of two lobes. The posterior lobe stores two hormones produced by the hypothalamus. In the anterior lobe at least 10 hormones are produced including one that regulates thyroid function. Also produced here are the female/male hormones which initiate reproduction of the egg/ sperm. The pituitary is also responsible for production of the growth hormone governing the maturity of the physical body.

Its relationship with the hypothalamus is essential for it is the hypothalamus which controls the pituitary secretions. The hypothalamus also controls body temperature, drives for hunger and thirst as well as the libido. Since messages traveling to and from the brain go through the hypothalamus, it coordinates activity in the nervous system with those in the endocrine system. The hypothalamus releases hormones stored in the posterior pituitary and "turn on" hormones which stimulate secretions by other endocrine glands from the anterior pituitary.

The seventh chakra's energy influences the pineal gland. This gland is cone shaped and is linked to altered states of consciousness. At this stage of evolution, scientists speculate that the pineal gland reaches its height of development at age seven. Scientists also believe it influences the endocrine system and the central nervous system although they are as yet unsure about the extent or nature of this influence.

Scientists believe that the pineal is related to reproduction and serves as an internal clock since it responds indirectly to light. When darkness moves to daylight, the pineal switches on secreting melatonin, a light-affected chemical relevant to pigment cells. The production of melatonin is triggered by exposure of the eyes to light. Melatonin causes blanching of the pigment cells of amphibians, but has no influence on mammalian pigment cells.

The pineal appears to inhibit the release of pituitary gonadotropins preventing precocious puberty. A chemical found in the brain and synthesized by the pineal has proven to be an agent which induces mystical states of consciousness. It has also been identified that melatonin is related to harmaline, a psychedelic drug processed from the Banisteriopsis vines of the Amazon and weakly linked to LSD. Harmaline has long been used by Indians to induce altered states of consciousness.

It is true that light produces excitation and de-excitation of electrons in an atom. As electrons circle in orbit they lose or gain energy by leaping from one orbit to another. Each leap is a quantum jump. When an electron jumps to a higher orbit it must absorb an amount of energy. When electrons move to lower orbits, back toward the nucleus, energy is released as a photon of light.

In the next chapter we will describe the ego chakra. This chakra is actually a system of energy recycling working directly with the major-minor and minor chakra areas of the physical body. These chakras form a minor chakra system insuring the continued availability of the physical body. Examples of major-minor chakra areas include the shoulder joints, elbows, wrists, hip joints, knees, and ankles. Minor chakra areas include the joints of the fingers and toes. These chakras also correspond to smaller nerve plexuses and sometimes coincide with acupuncture points not associated with the major chakra system. When the major-minor and minor chakra areas are working properly, the physical body maintains its strength, resiliency, and vitality. Energy can flow smoothly throughout the system without disruption. The maintenance of these chakras is the primary reason movement of the body or physical exercise is important.

The movement of the body alone is insufficient for stimulating the major-minor and minor chakras into action. In fact, physical exercise performed with little mental attention or by forcing of the body to go past its limits repeatedly will result in injury or body breakdown. These cause a distortion and misuse of major-minor and minor chakra energies resulting in painful disorders such as tennis elbow or football knee or in the case of professional athletes the early breakdown of the body's ability to continue to rebound. Students versed in the connection of mind-body will use visualization, proper breathing, and energizing-relaxing principles during physical exertion for maximum efficiency in causing these chakras to function. When the chakras are consistent in their motion, energy is continually resupplied to insure longevity in body functioning enabling the thinker a viable vehicle for learning throughout physical life.

Proper chakra function assures proper physical functioning and longevity. When the inner workings of the chakras are known we can begin influencing their function. By noting the physical manifestation of chakra energies we can readily trace the cause for harmonious or disharmonious function back to its source in the mental attitude. When symptomatic relief of a disorder can be supported by a mental attitude adjustment, health is restored and perpetuated. In this way the body becomes a measure of how productively we are using consciousness. When we love Self, others, and life, promoting progressive and positive ways of thinking, our physical bodies are stronger and healthier. When we fail to see the beauty and opportunity in life, filling our minds with negativity such as blame, cynicism or other forms of fear, our physical body weakens eventually become diseased.

A healthy physical body is an asset for pursuing the expansion of consciousness. Because mental attitudes of wholeness and productivity produce good physical health, this is desirable for anyone who wants to achieve the mystical states raising the Kundalini brings. When chakras function at their optimum rate, energy moves easily from the mind to the body freeing each to fulfill their function and purpose. You can learn to directly influence the movement of each chakra through directed mental perception. For this reason we will examine each chakra in light of the predominant quality of thinking which governs its function. By learning these keys to consciousness and integrating them into your own thinking, you will accelerate your readiness to raise the Kundalini. You will find when you develop the consciousness underlying chakra function, you can more easily direct these energies thus producing the expansion of consciousness characteristic of the Kundalini experience.

The Ten Chakras

To initiate the intentional use of the powerful Kundalini energy requires previous experience in the inner levels of consciousness for the purpose of enlightenment. Chakras return the energy you have used in the creation of your desires back to the inner levels of consciousness. It is like watering parched earth, for it restores their fertility in preparation for the drawing of energy that occurs when the Kundalini is stimulated into action. Knowing how the chakras function, why they function the way they do, and what relationship they have with consciousness will assist you in manifesting your desire to become familiar with the Self mastery wielding Kundalini can bring.

Familiarity with the chakra energies is more than a prerequisite for one who desires to utilize the Kundalini. Knowing how the chakras function gives you control of creative energies. It enables you to replenish the inner level energies used during your visualization endeavors. Depletion causes mental and physical fatigue interfering with the reproduction of your desires in your subconscious mind. Knowing why the chakras function enables you to evaluate your mental strengths and weaknesses. This information frees you to improve the quality of your life, mentally, emotionally and physically. It also paves the way for the development of the transcendent consciousness use of the Kundalini will bring.

During his physical existence, Man requires physical rest and sleep. This has been apparent throughout history and in more recent times has become widely accepted through case studies of the effects of sleep deprivation. When man is deprived of sleep his ability to concentrate wanes proportionate to the time elapsing from his last restful state. Continuing without sleep leads to disorientation, aberrant thinking, animalistic behavior, and eventually will cause death. The reason for this begins long before the physical effects of the deprivation are experienced.

For most, the only opportunity for the energies to be reestablished in the mind occurs during sleep when the attention is fully removed from the physical sensations and the conscious mind is at rest. During these periods two major experiences occur within the inner levels of consciousness. One is the communication from the inner, subconscious mind to the outer, conscious mind in the form of dreams, and the second is the rejuvenation of energy in the mind through energy transformers known as chakras.

Because the conscious mind is at rest during sleep, no thoughts are being produced during this time. No habits are being called into action. No commands for body movement are given. The inner mind is free to perform its duty and function unencumbered by any conscious desire or limitation. This is the time the inner mind can utilize the chakras to replenish energies depleted during the waking state. During sleep, there is no draining of energies from any chakra since the conscious mind is inactive. As the chakras return used energy back into the inner levels, energy reserves are restored preparing the inner mind for the next day's conscious commands for experience. Even when there is no awareness of the inner mechanism of re-energizing the mind, sleeping is the one way you have to insure this inner rejuvenation.

When you fail to release your conscious attention from the physical, whether from a physical stimulus such as pain or a mental stimulus such as worry, you toss and turn, awakening to find yourself as tired as when you laid down to sleep. Because you kept a part of your attention in the physical level of consciousness, you have not allowed the replenishing of your energies to occur. In addition to other reasons you may have, you can now see how learning to mentally direct relaxation of your mind and body is important to your health and welfare. This state of relaxation is also important to the healing process and is why sleeping is a natural reaction to dis-ease. Again, when the conscious mind is at rest, the inner mind can work to reestablish balance in energies which will promote healing in the mind and body.

These natural functions -- sleep, re-energizing, and healing -- of the inner mind work under the guidance of Universal Law, seeking to establish harmony and balance. These natural functions can be brought under the direction of your intelligence, thereby functioning at your command. Under the instruction and guidance of someone who has studied and applied knowledge of these chakra centers, you can become familiar with these etheric energy transformers and learn how to cause replenishing at will. In this way, what for most is only a subconscious function becomes a part of conscious awareness and control. This contributes not only to the health of your physical body but brings the state of your emotional, mental, and spiritual health under the dominion of your conscious awareness.

There are seven major energy centers which correspond to physical energies in the body. Cosmic energy enters the human body through the medulla oblongota where it becomes the life force for the body. In the medulla oblongota strands of nerves cross to form a pyramid shape in the brain stem located in the upper portion of the spinal column. From this point of intake of cosmic energy, the life force is separated into four branches. One of these is the chakra flow of energy.

Because everything created in mind eventually finds a physical manifestation, the chakras correspond to physical energy centers. The physical points react to the amount and quality of energy flowing through its relative chakra center. When the energy is depleted, that part of the body will be sluggish in performing its function. For instance, when the Root Chakra is sluggish, disorders in the reproductive system will begin to appear. The quality of thinking causes the sluggishness in the energy supply that eventually becomes apparent as disease. This depletion of energy will determine the type of disorder that appears, its duration, and the seriousness of its condition. When the chakras are operating in the optimum of their capacity, the corresponding part of the body will be resilient. For instance, an "iron stomach" is characteristic of a well-functioning Solar Plexus chakra.

      Chakras are not causal agents, but they do have a duty and function to perform that enables you, the thinker, to experience life fully. Each individual chakra's purpose for existence is based upon the area of consciousness it replenishes. How that purpose is being manifested by the creative intelligence will determine how well the chakra is allowed to perform its duty and function. Thus the quality of thought associated with each center is the most important and dominant factor in its proper function. By becoming acquainted with the quality of thought and accelerating your understanding of that quality in your every day awareness, you will influence each chakra to perform its duty. You will also become familiar with the expansion of consciousness which precedes and accompanies stimulation of the Kundalini.

The ego chakra

"Self" consciousness begins with an awareness of the me in man which expresses itself in what we know as ego. Ego is what motivates every thought and statement you have which includes the word "I". It describes our separate existence and embodies what we have become. The expression of ego in the physical is termed the conscious ego, although this sense of "I" may be found in all levels of consciousness. The conscious ego has a duty and function. This is most aptly described as a motivating force for it is the ego that sustains movement in our existence even when our consciousness is asleep.

When the soul enters a physical body for a lifetime of learning, the evidence of self consciousness quickly makes itself known. Children in the same family who have the advantages of the same general environment and are exposed to similar experiences will demonstrate their uniqueness from the time of birth. One is shy and observant, another precocious and creative, another hyperactive and emotional, while another is thoughtful and precise. Throughout the years of youth, the soul begins to express its understanding, and lack of it, through the consciousness of the conscious "I" creating the differences in self expression. Presented with the same experience, such as performing before an audience, the shy child might say "I am scared"; the precocious child, "I want to be first"; the hyperactive child, "I don't want to"; the thoughtful child, "I need more practice." Each are beginning to form patterns of identity that will determine later choices in life.

The expression of "I" is formed through a duality. Early training of this new conscious mind furthers the development of

"I" as the child ages. Parental expectation and instruction forms one part of this duality. When the child is expected to excel and offered the means of discipline required for excellence, the "I" rapidly gains strength displaying exceptional skill in learning and the confidence it brings. When the child is expected to bend to authoritarian rule and compromise in order to fit in, the "I" develops in a weakened condition unsure of its individual importance and lacking in self esteem.

The world is filled with stories of great adults who have enjoyed the benefits of strong and purposeful parenting in their early years as well as those who have surpassed less desirable beginnings of inattentive and deficient parenting. In a similar way, children sharing the same upbringing can demonstrate widely diverse productivity as adults. One can evolve into a dynamic, creative being influencing many toward the common good, while another sinks into troubling negativity becoming a burden to others. Thus the duality of the expression of "I" becomes apparent.

These elements of opposition occur because we are dual in nature. Once incarned, we are conscious beings responding and reacting to stimuli in our environment. We are also spiritual beings. The permanent part of self resides in the soul which chooses incarnation. This soul or subconscious mind holds the benefits of many lifetimes of learning and seeks expression through the "I" consciousness. Perhaps most apparent in the advent of a child prodigy, these understandings cannot be denied and will eventually become known in the building and fashioning of what we term personality.

The conscious ego reacts to physical stimuli. The information stored in the brain quickly becomes available for use as memory. The ego's action is to draw upon this stored information to motivate the conscious mind to perform its duty of reasoning. When a soul possesses an understanding of sound and receives encouragement from his environment to express this understanding we find a child who exhibits musical talent. When a physical stimulus is received, such as listening to the works of Mozart or watching the genius of Horowitz, the ego receives this stimulus saying "I can do that!" This motivates the conscious mind into action that will propel the learning, study, and practice to achieve. How many minds have received the stimulus of a Wilt Chamberlain or a Michael Jordan and responded with an "I can" motivation that leads them to excellence on the basketball court?

Because the ego only reacts to stimuli by drawing upon what is already stored in the brain, it does not determine productive or destructive motivation. This judgement is left to the conscious mind. If the brain has been filled with self-defeating concepts, these will be stimulated into action through memory. For instance, if a child seems to lack musical talent and he is instructed that he will never be able to play the piano whenever he is presented with the opportunity to learn, the ego will receive this stimulus saying "I'll never be able to do that" or "I'll never be as good as". It is still in the hands of the conscious mind to determine if the "I" will remain in this limited condition, giving up before even investigating the truth or fallacy of this self concept, or if the "I" will be reevaluated by recognizing the need and forming a desire to learn and excel. The former illustrates an individual who is ego motivated only. The latter describes the individual who has decided to become desire motivated. When the conscious mind learns to use the ego to its benefit it leaves previously formed limitations behind and begins to take control of the "I" promoting self development and awareness.

When we are ego motivated we are entrapped in our senses. We find ourselves at the mercy of what has been previously learned about who we are. Too many people live in this kind of stagnant existence, never realizing who they are, why they exist, or what they are here to do. They either follow the pattern they have seen others set, being only a follower, and killing awareness of their individual spirit with negative concepts of worthlessness; or they rebel against the limits and negativity they see around them, fighting against themselves and blaming others without ever identifying a solution to the problems they disdain. Many boast of their ability to remain the same, as if change automatically indicates something wrong or evil. To live a productive and purposeful existence is to be willing to change and evolve your "I" through the expansion of consciousness.

As we develop conscious awareness and control of the ego, we realize we are one part of a greater whole. We move beyond any limits of our "I", examining and evaluating how we respond in our conscious thinking to who we have become, who we are, and who we will be. Our thinking begins to recognize the needs of a developing mind, putting the ego into perspective. As this occurs we find the way we think about ourselves and others evolves. We realize we are unique and we seek ways to aid others by manifesting our specialness.

How we understand "I" of Self determines how the ego chakra will function. When we are changing, growing and learning, the major-minor and minor chakra system functions well by maintaining and rejuvenating the physical body so we have a physical vehicle with which to express our individuality. This major-minor chakra system exists throughout the body. Although these centers return used mental energy, their primary function is to return used physical energy for the purpose of maintaining the physical strength, dexterity, and vitality. Most of these energy transformers are found in joint areas. Major-minor chakras can be found at hinge joint areas such as the elbow and ball-and-socket joints such as the hip. They are also located in the palms of the hands, and these areas can be a site of drawing in cosmic energy or projecting it outward. Minor chakra areas include saddle joint and plane joint areas such as those found in the hand. As most people age, the sutures of the skull lose their flexibility. No matter how old the physical body, the need remains for the skull to breathe. When energy is returned to the suture areas flexibility is restored.

The efficiency and effectiveness of our physical body is important, for a healthy body assists the mind in being prepared to take advantage of learning experiences. It is important to the expression of the "I" that the body respond to its commands. The athlete expects the body to respond with strength and resilience. Someone who believes they are not pretty expects the body to

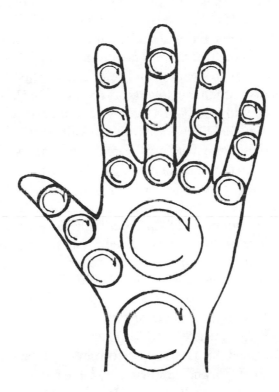

Major-Minor and Minor
Chakras of the Hand

reflect their concept of what is ugly. When you want to pick up something, you expect your body to move in specific ways to accomplish your mental desire.

One of the most obvious ways the functioning of this minor chakra system can be seen concerns the aging of the physical body. Scientists have studied the mysteries of aging for centuries concluding that there is no physically apparent reason for the human body to wear out and deteriorate. This is verified with the advent of organ transplants. A sixty year old kidney can be transplanted into a body of a twenty year old and continue to function for sixty more years making that kidney 100 years old. The answer to this scientific mystery lies not in physics, rather it is found in the exploration of metaphysics, or what lies beyond the physical laws of nature.

As the "I" continues to evolve throughout a lifetime, the chakra energies continue to function well causing the major minor and minor areas of energy to continue to feed the body. When this occurs we find people in their seventies, eighties, nineties who continue to enjoy the benefits of learning in the physical. Actor and comedian George Burns is an excellent and widely known example of agelessness. When seventy-one year old actor Jack Palance accepted his Oscar in 1992, he demonstrated his physical "fitness" by performing one handed push-ups to an astounded and admiring audience throughout the world. He even addressed the need to elevate group consciousness to understand that physical age, far from being a limitation, is an asset to be respected and used. It is true that physical fitness follows mental fitness. When the mind is fit in its ability and willingness to learn, no matter how long it has existed physically, the body will reflect this fitness.

As we learn to respectfully use the "I" consciousness, accepting the ego for what it is, we can fashion our own destiny with awareness and turn our attention inward toward the expansion of consciousness that awaits us.

Since the major-minor and minor chakra centers keep energy flowing through the physical body, physical movement will assist in maintaining their function. Mentally image cosmic energy entering into your body through the medulla oblongata at the base of your skull. Visualize this energy as a stream of light entering your body and traveling throughout to all extremities flooding your body with life force. While visualizing a particular area of the body, gently stretch that area by tensing and then relaxing the muscles. Repetitions will assist the minor chakras in performing their function keeping the body fit and full of vitality. Mental activity combined with physical action will stimulate these chakra centers to return the energy you have used in physical exertion throughout your day's experiences.

The Root Chakra

The Root Chakra derives its name from the Icelandic *rot* which is connected with the Latin *radix* meaning that part of a plant which fixes itself in the earth and by means of its radicles imbibes nutriment. The Root Chakra fixes itself in the physical, earthly environment from which it receives nutrients for the soul in the form of experiences. With the movement of this chakra, we find the physical, material manifestation of thought. To build our self concept, conscious thinking must occur. We must be willing to identify the needs of the Self in order to know the identity of Self. This is so whether we are speaking of the individual, the stars and planets, or subatomic particles.

The Root Chakra is traditionally seen as the first chakra because it forms the foundation or base for the raising of the Kundalini energy. It is the first of seven energy transformers required for the continual functioning of man as a thinker. The relationship of the chakra system to the use of Kundalini is brought to light by familiarity with these energy transformers as vehicles for the movement of prana through our consciousness.

With each individual chakra there is a quality of thought which sets it into motion and governs its continual function. Because this is part of the inner makeup of man as a thinker and because this causal force remains unconscious to most we will refer to this in our description of the quality of each chakra as the result of instinct. We have discussed the instinctual action of the Ego chakra by describing it as the "I" chakra.

Instinctually, the Root Chakra can be termed the *chakra of needs*. The quality of thinking governing its action is the drive for Self Autonomy. By being equipped to shape the concept of self, we are insured of the awareness of identity or who we are separate from what is around us. We have awareness that we need the air to breathe but we are separate from the air, that we need nutrients for the body to exist but we are separate from the food we eat, that we need stable external conditions of temperature and climate but we are separate from the weather. Our common needs become apparent in those which insure the continuation of our physical existence. This universality in experience arises in the need for rest, warmth, shelter, and in the form of hunger. Responding to these needs insures our individual physical existence and also lays the foundation for the continuation of our species.

During the early evolution of Reasoning Man, thinking was dominated by the fulfillment of these needs for survival. In response to his constantly changing environment which posed threats to his existence, man found constant stimuli to think and act quickly effecting solutions to the problems of food scarcity, untamed wildlife, and inclement weather. Responding to these needs led to the advances of early technology in producing fire, the wheel and lever, planting and irrigation, and a host of creative endeavors considered primitive by many but so essential to the progress of mankind and still widespread in the world today.

As the conscious mind and physical body evolve, the needs for physical survival occupy less and less of man's thinking time. This is apparent in the more technologically advanced societies. For those living in the United States, needs for physical survival and comfort are met through cooperative ventures thus ensuring the continuation of the individual and society as a whole. The means exists for anyone to meet their physical needs through using their talents and skills in exchange for the services that provide food, shelter, and clothing. This frees the mind to explore its existence beyond physical boundaries elevating awareness to more spiritual needs. It is the pursuit of these spiritual needs that leads man to his greatest creative endeavors.

The Root Chakra is often associated with creativity. More appropriately, it is the beginning of awareness as a creative being. With the Root Chakra, Self perpetuation becomes the means for asserting autonomy. As we expand in our recognition of what is needed for our existence we become aware that our inner needs will be met by using our creativity to further relationships with our environment. To create we need more than the physical materials, we require the stimulus derived from interaction with other creative beings, with peers. As we recognize our autonomy we also recognize our own duality and thus become aware of our physical sexuality. Sexuality becomes the sacred union through celebration of differences recognized through our separateness. Our need to produce new life forms separate from the Self shows itself in the sexual urge to mate and produce offspring.

Through sex and reproduction of the species families are formed which became the seed for social structures. Historically, man has evolved through agricultural societies into nomadic tribes into the formation of cities which eventually have become countries. The need for cooperation is apparent throughout man's evolution finding its expression in one individual joining with another or with many others. The security gained through the continuation of structure be it the DNA structure for your body or a system of government for your country frees your creativity rather than limiting it for even these structures are malleable as needs in consciousness become known.

The duality manifested in sexuality also becomes apparent in a spiritual sense through our need to restore, renew, and reproduce. It exists in all forms and pervades consciousness. The word Father is from the Latin *pater* meaning pattern and the word Mother is from *mater* meaning matter. Every act of creation is the forming of a pattern in the matter of mind.

The duality signified by yin and yang describes the two complementary fundamental principles found in all things, beings, events, and periods of time. They are universal by their nature. Yin is the negative, the earth, femininity, darkness, represented by a broken line. Yang is the positive, the sky, masculine, brightness, symbolized in an unbroken line. These two principles represent the polarization constantly attracted to one another to unify, blend and merge producing creation. The Eastern symbol of the yin and yang is a circle symmetrically divided by a "s" shaped curved line. Half of the circle is dark signifying the yin and half is light symbolizing yang. The light section contains a singular dot symbolizing the need for receptivity to exist in order for aggressiveness to be stimulated into action. This is the universal need. The yin-yang symbol represents the autonomy and the interdependency of the two principles, constantly influencing each other, never hostile. Always attracted by and to one another in order to produce wholeness, the aggressive and receptive principles epitomize need for they require one another for creation.

Creativity is inherent in every part of nature, finding its greatest challenge and manifestation through man's thinking capabilities. The greatest need for human man is to create. The Root Chakra transforms the energy we use in creating, returning it back into specific areas in mind, so we will have a continual supply of energy for future creative endeavors. When its energy is well used, the Root Chakra becomes a seat of creativity through which we can experience the childlike wonder and excitement of our manifest universe.

Far beyond providing the energy the conscious mind requires for the manifestation of physical conditions desired, the Root Chakra energy finds its highest use by one who recognizes the need to know Self as a Creator. Such a one is aware of the inner urge which initiated and formed this chakra center. By calling upon the creative abilities to fulfill a higher purpose of maturing the identity of the whole Self, the conscious mind breaks free of limitation and the expansion of consciousness begins.

Moving beyond the goals that can be set to fulfill apparent needs, the conscious mind finds its expansion of consciousness by becoming purposeful. To have purposes for your ideals lifts your awareness beyond physical attainment and into the realms of Self development and exploration. Purpose is how the actions of attaining a goal will impact your Self concept, how it will alter your identity. When your thoughts are spiritual in nature, the attainment of physical needs brings spiritual unfoldment.

In the Sanskrit language, the Root Chakra is known as Muldhara. *Mula* means root and *adhara* means support. The recognition of Self as a Spiritual entity is the origin of the foundation for your existence. As manifested in the ethers, the Root Chakra is symbolized by a four petal lotus. It is not by chance that the number four signifies stability and can be found throughout our existence. Four is the number of the cardinal directions: north, west, south, and east. There are four elements: earth, water, fire, and air. The seasons are divided into four: winter, spring, summer, and fall. There are four stages of life: infancy, adolescence, adulthood, and old age.

The Root Chakra reflects the creative foundation for building consciousness. The productive use of this chakra results in transforming concepts of Self Identity. The more balanced an individual is in his or her understanding and use of the aggressive and receptive qualities, the more he or she will draw upon this energy. Such a one is assertive and cooperative during the same time. He is acquainted with the actions of the emotions. He realizes the word *emotion* describes the consciousness it directs well. From the Latin *movere* meaning to move and *e* meaning out, the purpose for emotion is to act in the inner, subconscious mind, and to react in the outer, conscious mind. The conscious mind cooperates with the manifesting desires moving from the inner mind into physical manifestation. The enlightened individual chooses to respond to his own creations, rather than reject, suppress, or deny them.

Where there is misuse of the Root Chakra energy you will find a denial of the needs of self. This is aptly manifested in the attitudes and action of the anorexic who denies the need for physical nourishment thus leading to the destruction of the physical body. However, procrastination on the fulfillment of needs is also characteristic of misuse of this energy as evidenced in wishful thinking or in the jealousy arising from coveting what another exhibits. This leads to poverty of spirit and flesh.

An attachment to the satisfying of the physical senses alone is another example of misusing of this chakra's energy. This feeds a dependency upon what is transient eventually breeding sorrow, despair, and anger when the coveted object no longer exists to fill our need. Attachment will produce eliminatory disorders characteristic of a depletion of Root Chakra energy. From the momentary irritation experienced during an electrical power failure to the more long-standing grief of the loss of a loved one, our emotional reactions are keys to be used to identify a lack of understanding in Self. Responding to this lack by coming to terms with and learning the lesson presented to us, produce the independence of creating anew.

Misuse of the Root Chakra can also manifest due to limited and restricted ideas concerning sexuality. When our thinking is bound by sexual taboos, the proper flow of energy is difficult to achieve and maintain. Refusing to respond to the sex the soul has chosen for learning retards the growth and development throughout a lifetime. Physically going through the motions of sexual activity, without thought or ideal, leads to a depletion of spirit and eventually can manifest in a weakening of the reproductive system. This can lead to debilitating venereal disease. Rejecting the soul's choice will produce denial of the masculine or feminine qualities and eventually breed disorders in the reproductive system. When the identity is seen as worthless in terms of the understanding of Self as a creative being and the sexual expression of Self, the body becomes weakened setting the stage for Acquired Immune Deficiency Syndrome.

Also characteristic of a misuse of this energy is an attitude of blame. When someone is looking for a scapegoat he will find one. Whether it is society, a close associate, or even the self, the person who looks for an excuse not to change can always discover someone or something in his way. This type of thinking breeds insecurity and promotes resentment toward our ability to have the kind of life we desire. This will produce imbalances in physical fertility. Learn to be a leader rather than a follower. Instead of passively waiting, make the kind of life you want.

Instead of bullying your way through life, give your Self a chance to receive from life's abundance.

By cooperating with the natural energy flows of the Root Chakra, we learn to perpetuate our creative ability which aids us in producing wholeness in mind and body. By using creativity daily, we perpetuate the manifestation of life experiences that can help us become whole. By responding to what we create in life, we cause this energy to recycle preparing us for future creation.

To cause this transformer to function properly, develop the attitudes of Self assertion and cooperation in fulfilling the needs of the Self. First, admit your needs. Release self-denial patterns of thought. Affirm your importance daily through thought and action. Do something just for your Self each day. Visit an old friend, treat your self to a movie, take a drive in the country, read a novel. Second, create and respond! Always have a creative project. Develop a hobby be it woodworking or playing a musical instrument. Write. Practice receiving the benefits of what you have created. Graciously accept compliments. Third, pursue Self discovery. Discover what you think about your sexual choice. Realize the possibilities of why you, the soul, may have chosen to be male or female. Fourth, practice visualization daily.

The Adrenal (Spleen) Chakra

The second energy transformer, the Adrenal Chakra, is also known in esoteric studies as the Spleen Chakra. Instinctually, this is the *chakra of desire*. The quality of thinking which governs its action can be described as Self reliance. Self Reliance occurs when we are aware of what we possess as a thinker and are willing to use what is at hand to produce what we desire. This can be seen in the ability to use resources in our everyday physical life. It also applies to the recognition of mental skills that can make our lives more efficient and more rewarding. By admitting the power of desire, we bring to ourselves the freedom creativity affords.

When the needs of Self are received and admitted by the conscious mind, the power of imagination becomes activated seeking ways to fill those needs. In this way we find the further development of man's identity as a creative being. When we are hungry we seek food, when we are lonely we seek companionship, when we are ignorant we seek education. When we find we are deficient in any area, we look for ways to become whole. This seeking is answered through the power of desire.

Desire finds its greatest accomplishment in the blending of creative imagination and a well developed will. Being the expression of the thinker in the physical, the conscious mind possesses three key abilities readily available for the production of desire. First it has information stored in the brain. When called into action by the thinker, this information becomes useable as what we call memory. By drawing on previous experiences, the conscious mind can call upon its creative ability of imagination to produce a new, improved image that reflects the filling of its need. This new, improved image is desire. For instance, seeing a young couple in love may stimulate our need for companionship. We can respond to our need in a variety of ways. We may choose to ignore the couple's passion, judging it as inappropriate or the failing of youth, thus denying our own need and cutting short our own creative ability. We may envy what we perceive as the closeness and rapport the couple enjoys, again stifling our awareness of our need and leaving ourselves lonely. We may observe with interest the couple's interaction, admitting our desire to experience the love, tenderness, and communication we see. This will stimulate our memory of previous associations we have had leading us to begin wondering "what if". This ability to conjure "what if" is the beginning of formulating our own desire for something we want to experience in our lives.

At this stage of evolution, our needs of physical survival have been transcended. For Reasoning Man physical survival is an indirect process. For instance, we obtain food from a store rather than needing to maintain a fire or guard our stockpile of food from predatory animals. Freed from survival consciousness, our attention is now free to include our inner emotional, mental, and spiritual needs. This opens the door for us to admit our desires.

For a compulsive thinker, awareness of the need for food will be quenched by whatever is at hand and readily available. For a thinker, this awareness stimulates the imagination to form a desire for what will satisfy the hunger. Depending upon the situation, you direct the means of fulfillment. You might imagine and create a delicious meal, or you might choose a cuisine from a myriad of fine restaurants. You might eat a piece of fruit or a candy bar, or you might elect to postpone eating until the next meal time. Through the acceptance and respect for your ability to separate your needs from your desires, you free your consciousness to respond intelligently through choice rather than limit your awareness with a have or have-not physical consciousness.

The effects of the have or have-not consciousness can be seen throughout existence and has been the impetus for every conflict, whether between neighbors or nations, man has known. When imagination is lacking, man relies upon what has been, becoming territorial. This can be seen in the jealousy and taking of another's possessions, in the defensiveness and squabble to keep "your" place in line, or in a nation's efforts to squelch new ideas. Man tries to keep conditions the same in a constantly changing world. By habitually holding on to what has been, he drains this chakra's energy through the denial of his desire.

Threats to the continuity of existence stimulate the adrenal glands to provide a burst energy of short duration. What begins as a desire to perpetuate and continue existence deteriorates into what is known as *fight or flight*. This instinctual reaction exists to maintain self possession in unexpected crises. As has often been noted, crises brings out the best or the worst in people. When a hurricane or earthquake strikes, heroes are born. Many respond by creatively helping one another to find safety, shelter and food while others react by selfishly grabbing for what will fill their own needs first, forgetting they are part of a community. Still, others may use the occasion to thieve. The difference between the hero and the thief lies in the consciousness of each. The heroes use the burst of energy to create desires in response to the needs at hand. The self-centered people react from habitual fear of losing what little they have. Both are the result of thinking patterns established long before the crisis arose.

Crisis thinking is characteristic of those who are unfamiliar with the energies of the Adrenal Chakra. The quality of thinking which governs its action is the drive for purpose. It demands the awareness of Self as a creative being above and beyond problem solving. Problem solving means the thinker has waited too long to display the creativity he possesses. We have waited to fail before we consider what will produce success, we have postponed pursuing health until we become ill, we have procrastinated on becoming wealthy before we learn how to invest our money, we have ignored indications of our intuitiveness leaving us trapped by the physical senses only. Although hindsight can be a great stimulus for learning, when it is the only way you learn you are still deaf, dumb, and blind to your inner needs. When inner needs are admitted, the imagination is activated for the fulfillment of those needs through the desire and creativity flourishes.

Adrenal Chakra energy is more productively used by someone who is imaginative. When you are creative in and with your life, this energy serves to give you sustaining power and the endurance necessary to create your desires. You are no longer a victim of life because you no longer require a crises to get you moving. By becoming familiar with your own desires, you cause movement in your life in the direction you desire. This is the true meaning of power. Power is not the result of being better, stronger, or smarter than someone else is, nor is it being richer or healthier than your neighbor. Power is your ability to be more than you were yesterday. It is the ability to cause change at will and this is the secret to being purposeful in your thoughts.

Your inner urge is to express your own creative power. When you realize everything in the universe is in perpetual motion, you can harmonize your thinking to include change. This opens your awareness to your power to influence motion. By merely existing, you influence everyone and everything around you. The people you live and work with, the type of car you drive, the home you keep, and the air you breathe are changed because you exist. Nothing is ever the same once you have entered into its realm of existence. In the same way, you are influenced by the existence of everything around you. A decision made by a president today can set into motion conditions that will affect the quality of your life. The burning of rain forests in South America can affect the climate where you live. An earthquake on the opposite side of the globe or solar flares can affect the quality of your life. To understand power and influence is to admit you are part of a much greater whole. What you can do as a part of that whole will either progress mankind forward in evolution or retard that progression.

The Sanskrit word describing the Adrenal Chakra is *Svadhisthana*. The root word *svad* means to sweeten what belongs to itself and *dhisthana* implies its actual place. This captures the essence of the parts in the whole for it describes the forces that act upon each other. By understanding Self possession, who we are, we can evolve our awareness of Self importance realizing our place in creation and our relationship with creation.

The Adrenal Chakra is often illustrated as having six petals. The form of six is six triangles. Pythagoreans recognized six as the midpoint between two and ten, one was not counted as a numeral. In China, six was associated with the influence called heaven. For the Christian six is sacred appearing in the six days of creation and in the 666 noted in Revelation. The hexagram formed the Seal of Solomon and the Star of David recognized the six-pointed star formed by two superimposed triangles. For the Hindu, six is the union of Yoni and the Linga, representing respectively the female and male sexual organs. The six occurs in Judaism, Christianity, Islam, and it underlies the India Yantra meaning a geometic representation. In alchemy the six represents the union of all opposites because it comprises the basic forms of the signs for elements.

When productively used, the Adrenal Chakra energies will assist you in realizing your personal power for you will become familiar with how creation impacts on Self. You will begin expecting abundance and prosperity to be part of your life. By constantly expanding your awareness of the resources open to you, you will grow in the Self reliance which draws upon this center's energy. You will know that to expect and have the best makes it easier to create and use.

One of the greatest misuses of this energy is the fear of losing creative ability thus being power-less. When potential desires are ignored or denied, the mind becomes fertile to the misuse of imagination. The greatest misuse of your ability to imagine makes itself known through your fears. For instance, you are working late. When you finally leave your place of employment, the parking lot seems desolate and is dimly lit. With your thoughts undirected by your intelligence, you begin to conjure images of danger - the very things you do not want. Fear is the result of imagining what you do not desire in your life.

By practicing fear again and again, you become a victim of your own imagination and you find yourself playing out the role of the victim in your life. You begin believing everyone is against you, when in truth you are your own worst enemy. Fear can stimulate the action of the adrenal glands to give you immediate power to ward off physical danger, but desire gives you sustaining power to experience the benefit of experiencing what you want in your life.

Many people become angry to disguise their fear. The metaphor of venting your spleen refers to a misuse of this energy. Anger can also arise from the have-not attitude. Instead of being jealous of someone else's use of power, realize what is missing is your own use of power. Tearing down what someone else has built cheapens your existence and destroys the quality of life for us all. Make understanding your goal replacing anger with productive Self empowerment.

Another misuse of this energy is trying to keep what you have rather than adding to it. This procrastination will lead to disorders in the eliminatory systems of the body, particularly the colon and kidneys. Repeatedly putting off the fulfillment of desires results in the backing up of waste in the large intestines. When you wait for a crisis to force you into action, you may begin having irritable bowel problems. The regret associated with a lifetime of procrastination will cause kidney disorders. So will a succession of "I shoulds". Instead of refusing to create your desires, begin embracing life experiences. Instead of looking for purpose as if it is something you have lost, realize and invoke your ability to make your thoughts, your actions, and your life purposeful. This will move you forward in life.

To use the Adrenal Chakra energies first, develop an image of Self reliance by responding as situations arise. Pursue learning skills to support your image. If you don't know how - learn to: cook, drive, balance a checkbook, make your bed, or read a map. Second, develop purposefulness. Take an inventory of your physical possessions. Discover what resources you have. When was the last time you wore that college sweatshirt, used that broken radio, or read those old magazines? Clean out your closet, attic, and garage. Make two piles. In one place all the things you will never use again. In the second place all the things you still want to use. Give away what you can from pile one and make a list of pile two items and how you will use them in the next six months. Third, play games of strategy. By strengthening memory, attention, and imagination you will develop the ability to create forward motion. This will replace dependency on crises. By training your mind to delineate cause and effect you will begin to see the whole picture of what is before you. You will also learn how to live in the present, to be here now.

The Solar Plexus Chakra

Instinctually the Solar Plexus Chakra, the third center, is the *chakra of attainment.* The quality of thinking governing its action can be described as Self Identity. The sense of self first evident in the expression of the ego is now refined and developed by the recognition of needs and the formulation of desires that will fill those needs. Much more than physical personality, Self identity is awareness of the duality of Self as Spiritual and physical, inner and outer. The constantly changing needs and desires as we move through life produce the image of who we are and provide the opportunity awareness of Self apart from those experiences. Thus the establishment of Self Identity comes by identification through separation.

Typically, man has developed by seeing people, countries, land, cultures, races, or periods of history as separate isolated building blocks coordinated through control rather than natural order. For instance, medical science treats the parts of body as separate ailing units rather than connections to a whole, working system. To offset one disorder, the chemical balance of the body is altered through the use of drugs as if the chemical will only affect the designated part of the body it is meant to balance. However, this is never the case, and the rest of the body is left to deal with the unbalancing effect the drug produces. These are medically termed "side effects", but too often they become primary effects to further disorders in the bodily system. When the ability for health through productive attitudes is realized the need for chemically altering the body state will become obsolete. When the imbalance in thinking is identified and corrected, the physical body will respond in a similar fashion.

The Solar Plexus Chakra energies are responsive to balance and imbalance. This is readily seen in physical body reactions to cold and heat or in the craving or avoidance of spicy foods. A quick trip on an elevator can "leave your stomach" on the tenth floor when the rest of your body has reached ground level. That slight feeling of queasiness is the imbalance of energies in the solar plexus. Likewise, this can be experienced in the nausea that may follow the receiving of emotionally upsetting news. The imbalance first occurs in the thinking processes, then is registered in how the energy of this chakra has been altered by either too little or too much energy.

As we move through life experiences, a strong sense of Self concept is established. The creativity begun with the Root Chakra and developed with the Adrenal Chakra has moved the thinker to collect experiences which form the awareness of what we possess. We realize we have thinking patterns, behavioral patterns, and their subsequent effects in our lifestyle for the purpose of creating balance in our lives. We seek balance in every part of our life. Work needs to be balanced with recreation, relationships need to be a process of giving and receiving, daydreams need to be balanced with night dreams, and perhaps most importantly our outer Self and inner Self need to become known so both can operate in a balanced fashion creating a whole Self. We realize we *have* in order to create an awareness of balance.

Through expressing the personal power born through purposeful thinking we now can experience the power in diversity. The strength of any group or organism depends on solidarity and solidarity is provided through unity. Unity is the result of our ability to combine and coordinate forces to create something new. In this way, we discover balance through separation, unification, and cooperation. On an individual scale these can be seen in every area of our lives; in a male uniting with a female to form a marriage and family, in a worker uniting with a company to provide a service, or in a nervous system uniting with other systems to form the functional human body. In order for the family, the business, or the body to be productive in its purpose for existence, individual creative power must be active. This is also true on a global scale. As a whole, we give creative power a direction for humanity.

The energies of the Solar Plexus Chakra become evident in our ability to connect, for it is connection which produces balance. The sense of belonging that arises in long term associations gives us a sense of the continuity in relationships. We realize we are not isolated in our separateness, rather we come to know our likenesses and our differences as the basis for unity. The word community includes the word "unity" for it symbolizes the coming together of the diverse for a common ideal. When this type of cooperation exists, there is a love for home, family, country, and the world.

Our ability to move our thinking beyond our own experiences depends upon how well we know ourselves as spiritual beings. This becomes an integral part of using the Solar Plexus Chakra energies productively for they respond readily to an individual's awareness of his own karmic indebtedness. *Karma* is a Sanskrit word meaning act or fate. The physical manifestation of the Universal Law of Cause and Effect, karma is most appropriately described as *indebtedness to Self*. It is sometimes referred to as the Law of Balance.

Often misunderstood, the working of karma in our lives insures the growth and maturity of our Selves as spiritual beings. One who is acquainted with its workings, knows that karma guides the experiences of unenlightened man. In our quest to become enlightened creators, an understanding of karma can accelerate our movement on the path of development. Karma is set into motion not by the actions we perform, as commonly thought; rather karma is set into motion by the intentions behind our actions. It is not the action of cutting with a knife that causes karma, it is the intention in the mind of the person wielding the knife. For instance, a robber may use a knife to wound and kill his awakened prey. The robber's intention is to steal and murder anyone who tries to thwart his mission. Yet, a doctor may use a knife in surgery which results in the death of his patient. The doctor's intention was to extend a life even though this did not transpire. Both the robber and the doctor used similar tools, with similar actions, but the intentions were radically different. Karmically, both are accountable for their intentions and both have produced experiences that can afford learning.

By becoming consciously aware of our karmic inden-
tures, we expand our perception of everyday physical experiences.
We become aware of the purpose for our experiences and free
our minds to live life fully. What was unknown becomes known.
Every situation in life whether consciously or unconsciously
produced becomes an opportunity to add understanding to the
soul. We understand why we keep having the same type of boss,
why someone marries the same type of person again and again,
why one person lives while another dies. Awareness of personal
karmic obligations are revealed in past lifetime research. Once
these obligations are recognized, we have a way to further our
understanding and use of Solar Plexus energies.

When we realize we exist in the physical for the purpose
of learning, the way we see our Selves and the world changes.
We know that there is more to life than what the physical senses
receive. We know that there is more to life than eating, sleeping,
working, mating, and dying. We begin reaching to include the
perspective of our soul. We seek this awakening through
spiritual endeavors. Some become acquainted with spirituality
through religious guidance and ceremony, others through good
works and community service, others through communing with
nature, and others through prayer and meditation. How well we
tune our attention to inner awareness of the soul will determine
the quality of the needs and desires we form in our lives. It will
also determine how well we respond to inner cravings by feeding
our soul.

With this enlightened awareness, we take greater care in
how we create our ideals and purposes. We move beyond the
physical limitations which are transient, and reach for what is
permanent in our experience. Here we discover that it is the
understandings we are able to glean from our physical experiences which are added to our soul. As we reach toward
understanding we achieve balance and fulfill the karmic indebtedness to our Self. We begin to take note of what is known and
made a part of the Self, and what has yet to be known. With this
knowledge we can move forward in our lives using the Solar
Plexus energies productively.

In Sanskrit the term for this chakra is *Manipura* meaning city of jewels. This aptly describes the value we can perceive when we become acquainted with the inner and outer selves. Leaving behind the limitations of the have and have-not, our attention now is focused upon the progression of desires that will fill the needs of our soul.

This chakra is illustrated with ten petals. Ten is the sum of the first four numbers: one, two, three, and four. It is considered a Holy number for it symbolizes wholeness with understanding. This shows in the decimal system as a return to unity or the highest level. In China, ten is associated with totality. In the Bible ten symbolizes this wholeness in the stories of the ten commandments, the ten Egyptian plagues, the ten virgins, and the ten lepers. To Pythagorus, ten was a sacred number. It was regarded as the sum, the source all things being personified as a god of harmony.

The Solar Plexus Chakra is used productively by someone who balances their personal power by empowering others. Being confident in Self Identity, he endeavors to unify others to work together as a unit toward a common good. The current awareness of ecology is an example of such an intention for it brings to the awareness the responsible use of power. This responsibility is the use of substances and return used energy, thus everything is useful and nothing is wasted.

The quality of openness is outstanding in one who uses this energy well. He is open to experience and the understanding it can afford. There is a calmness in such a person, even during times of stress. Fortified by empathy, he transcends "me" concerns which permits him to connect with others and feel the contentment associated with connection.

When you believe you are just a number in society rather than an individual, you lose sight of your identity. This causes imbalance in your thinking, disrupting the energies of the Solar Plexus. When isolation occurs you lose the concept of power within. You function in an alienated job to receive a salary often doing work you resent, rather than to assist in the ideals of the company and add to your own learning. When these types of attitudes rule you will find the beginning of stomach disorders. If you lose sight of your reason to live, depletion of Solar Plexus energies will become apparent in a degeneration of the liver.

An excessive drive to be in power, to dominate and control, stems from insecurity in Self identity and will result in imbalances in the pancreas. Most often this will appear as diabetes for these thinking patterns lead to unbalancing thoughts that one must take what is wanted rather than create what is wanted. This type of selfishness can also manifest as a need to be noticed, constantly demanding or taking other's attention eventually producing hypoglycemia in the body. Characteristic of a sluggish Solar Plexus Chakra is an "I can't" attitude. Giving up before you even start is the fastest way to limit your learning. Try giving up your limitation!

By establishing your sense of identity as a soul as well as a physical being, you free your mind to pursue the highest learning available. This brings confidence in who you are and your ability to create what you want with any conditions you experience. As a result, you build security within, and what you gain inwardly as a soul is yours permanently to call into action anytime, anywhere, with anyone.

To stimulate the action of the Solar Plexus Chakra, first, recall the games you played as a child. Remember who you pretended to be when you were a child. The games you played, particularly when you were alone from the ages of one to seven, can reveal your soul's intention for this lifetime. Write down what you remember. Ask your parents or siblings if they remember the roles you played. How have you cooperated with these dreams of the soul? Second, become aware of your conscious mind's intentions. At the end of each day review your experiences. Were your thoughts and actions aligned? Join a club or organization whose ideals you believe in and support. Give your time and energy to these ideals adding your creative efforts to those of others. Third, begin recording and deciphering your nighttime dreams.

The Heart Chakra

Instinctually, the Heart Chakra is the *chakra of commitment*. The quality of thinking governing its action is Self Acceptance. Here the relativity of experience and understanding is explored adding an expansive quality to the soul's learning. Characteristic thinking affecting this energy involves our relationships to our environment, the people, places, and things in our lives. It now becomes increasingly important that our thinking include others. Our willingness to commit ourselves in thought and action brings the fulfillment of longevity in our relationships. By completing any action, mental or physical, which we initiate we come to understand the benefits of commitment in our life and our ability to respond is enhanced. We begin to unite the conscious mind and the subconscious mind toward common endeavors producing a sense of wholeness in the way we know our Selves and our world.

With the Heart Chakra we easily move beyond learning from our physical experiences only. Now we can learn through experiences stored not only in the brain's memory but also in the permanent memory of the soul. This frees us to integrate information and understanding into our consciousness to influence our actions for the growth of Self and others. As reasoning is heightened, we develop foresight enabling us to create more completely the ideals we hold. Far beyond the setting of physical goals to accomplish, ideals incorporate the meaning of desires. When ideals are created, individual values reach to unite with universal values and thus enhance the quality of life for everyone.

For this reason, the Heart Chakra is associated with the emanation of love toward everything we encounter. Far beyond the limits of the emotional reaction of what we term love, this is an awareness of good will toward all. Emotional love finds its root in the temporary conditions of likes and dislikes. We attach this love to the objects of our affection. This object-oriented love is a passion stimulated and dictated by the presence of a person, place, or thing. It is conditional based upon willingness of that object to continue giving what we find pleasurable. Conditional love says, "I will love you as long as you...." When the object's giving ceases, the love vanishes, or when the object is no longer present the conditional love finds itself empty in its absence.

Having a dual nature, this type of love can also manifest as an unconditional love. Here the attachment of the likes overrules sound judgement, leaving its perpetrator in undesirable conditions. Unconditional love says "I will love you no matter what..." Many people remain in destructive relationships from this misunderstanding of love. For whatever reason, the past (he wasn't always this way), the present (she's wonderful when she's off the drugs), or the future (when the children get older), this type of person makes the self a victim by choice. To elevate the awareness of love, is to use developed reasoning skills to transcend the duality of likes and dislikes and enter the world of understanding.

Heart Chakra energies flow from love that is a spiritual concern for well-being, not only of our Selves but for all of creation. A parent disciplines a child so the child may learn a lesson he willfully wants to avoid. Love is the incentive, for without love the parent would have no vision for the child's safety and learning. A friend is truthful because he can see we are making a mistake in thought or action. A child cares for a puppy because he knows the young animal needs assistance. These expressions of love come from a respect and acceptance of our place in creation.

By using the Heart Chakra energies, we discover peace in the fulfillment of our needs and desires. We come to accept our ability to create as the means for inner and outer harmony.

Through Self Acceptance we can freely admit we are creators of our lives. We leave behind self condemnation for past mistakes as we reach toward different ways of thinking that will resolve those errors in judgement and bring to the self an understanding of cause. We leave behind worry and anxiety confident in our ability to create a future we want to live. We leave behind ideas of superiority and inferiority, no longer gauging our sense of well-being on what someone else is, does, or has. Now our sense of security arises from the freedom to evaluate ourselves by the changes we have made in our Selves. What becomes important is how we are different from the person we were yesterday, and how we will become the person we want to be tomorrow.

Love frees the mind and heart to respond generously to life's experiences. Understanding those experiences births a new way of viewing responsibility. Unfortunately, few people know the secret of responsibility. Taught by elders the necessity of being responsible often the purpose and meaning are lost and left unknown. People tend to value responsibility but view it as a trap and a burden of adulthood. In reality, it is our ability to respond to anyone, at any time, anywhere that gives us freedom. When we can be who we want to be whether with kings or paupers, at work or at play, at home or in a foreign land, with strangers or our dearest loved ones, we truly know the meaning of freedom.

Many falsely hold onto the idea that escaping responsibility will produce freedom. They think a vacation will give them freedom, or a marital separation, or sending the kids to camp. Upon return from such short-term escapades the same situation awaits us. Even if we quit our job, divorce our spouse, and give up custody of our children, sooner or later we will find similar reactions to a new set of people. This is the manifestation of karma in our lives because karma insures we have a way to understand our experiences. By enhancing our ability to respond, we multiply the open avenues for greater understanding and unlock doors to understandings we already possess.

The more we understand cause, the more compassion we have to offer others. By giving deep consideration and resolving the questions of meaning in life -- why is one person born in a healthy body while another is sickly, why do children die an early untimely death, is there a God, a heaven, a hell -- we expand our awareness of who we are and our relationship with creation. The ability to create questions, seek resolution, and achieve points of understand increases the sense of permanent connection with all life forms. We realize all of creation is in a process of growth and we grow in our respect for the forces of the Universe which guide that evolution. No one is a stranger. No land is foreign. No belief is unworthy of consideration.

The Heart Chakra energies also respond to what can be termed affinity. Here the principles of attraction become acutely evident. In the maturation of our creative ability, when our own subconscious mind does not have what it needs to fulfill our desires, it will reach out to other subconscious minds with similar conscious commands. In this way, we are drawn toward certain people, places, and things for the fulfillment of our desires. When this occurs we find ourselves at the right place, at the right time, with the right people. To the untrained mind it seems like magic or a great deal of good luck. Those who have studied and applied metaphysical principles understand the powers of attraction, whether in the chemical affinity of two molecules of hydrogen and one of water or in the attraction between people because each has something the other wants. By assisting in the manifestation of ideals, the Heart Chakra energy gives us a way to understand the experiences produced by our directed creative power.

The Sanskrit word describing this center is *Anahata*. *Anahata* is the sound made without any two things striking. The unity produced through the balance of duality produces a vibratory pattern from the blending of what was two into one. It is organization with purpose be it oneness in the many parts of Self or community of many unique individuals.

This chakra is illustrated by twelve petals. Twelve was the fundamental number of the duo-decimal system used by Babylonians. It is a symbol of spacio-temporal fulfillment signifying wholeness. Twelve is significant in astronomy for there are twelve signs of the zodiac and in the measurement of time - twelve months or twelve hours in the day and twelve hours in the night. In the <u>Bible</u> twelve symbolizes mastery of creation evidenced in the twelve sons of Jacob, the twelve tribes of Israel, the number of gems on the breastplate of the Jewish high priest, the number of apostles, and the number of gates of Heavenly Jerusalem. The form of the twelve is comprised of three squares or four triangles.

When the Heart Chakra energies are productively used, we have a sense of our connectedness. We are prone to volunteer our time and effort in aiding others. We act upon our ideals to make the world a better place to live. Our attention is directed toward understanding in life rather than on temporary sense gratification and physical accomplishment. We understand the meaning of knowing something *by heart* for to commit knowledge to memory is to strive to commit the self to what is permanent. Self respect naturally leads to respecting others and a universal sense of compassion and love influences our thoughts and actions. Not surprisingly, it is compassion which stimulates the innate potential for healing. Being free from prejudice, the mind is open to new people and places embracing the wonder in life.

When the mind is closed by judgmental attitudes the Heart Chakra energies are stifled. Pre-judging ourselves or others leaves little room for learning and growth. Instead of benefitting from previous experience, memories become barriers to surmount. This leads to defensive attitudes of misdirected protection of what we have yet to understand. When we cannot explain what we think or why we think the way we do, we become defensive. Our Self concept deteriorates under a cloak of self righteousness. We begin viewing others as enemies, rejecting us for who we are, when in reality we are promoting self-rejection by refusing to develop a productive Self image. This type of defensiveness will erode the immunological systems of the body causing susceptibility to bacteria and viral conditions. If the thinking is perpetuated over time, the body can become sufficiently weakened to produce disease such as leukemia, lymphoma, or AIDS.

When an individual is seized by competitive thoughts, constantly looking for ways to best someone else, heart and circulatory disease will become apparent. Eventually, the internal pressure of trying to keep up with others will produce hardening of the arteries or restrictions in the functioning of the heart. Someone who tries to "look good" when he really doubts his own capability will misuse Heart Chakra energies leading to imbalances in blood pressure or arrhythmia.

When the individual is fighting his own concepts of love he begins to feel trapped by the conditions he places on love or the conditions others place upon love. This battle steals the vitality of the body by affecting the respiratory system and can appear in the form of asthma or sinus disorders. By continuing inner conflict, lung disorders will manifest in the body.

To stimulate the action of the Heart Chakra, first, complete what you start! How many projects do you have that are "on hold"? Follow through. Pay extra on your car payments, work on that partially refinished room, send out those resumes, either get married or let the relationship go. Second, find the Real You. Drop the role playing. Be open to others giving both of you a chance to release prejudices. Respond from within instead of how you think you'll look to others. What you want others to be, be that your Self. Set your own expectations and live up to your ideals. Third, learn a form of meditation that will enable you to practice expectancy.

The Throat Chakra

Instinctually, the Throat Chakra is the *chakra of expression*. The quality of thinking that governs this center is Self Awareness. Self awareness can be described as the use of mental attention to integrate perceptions of the world around us and the world within us. As the attention is directed toward the information received from the five physical senses we are able to produce awareness of our relationship with our environment. As our attention becomes singular and undivided we are able to possess recognition and awareness of our inner environment. We have investigated the movement of our ability to create as evidenced in the directing thoughts of the four lower chakras. Now we reach the point where the desire to communicate our perception of the world is possible. We find we have a desire to establish a rapport or a connection with others, and this is most easily facilitated through communication.

The qualities of the Throat Chakra center energies offer the opportunity for a rhythmic connection between the listener and the speaker. The communication of our thoughts through speech enables us to transcend our own personal Self and project those thoughts to others just as a telephone enables us to communicate from one physical location to someone at any location on the earth at will. More importantly, as we communicate we have an opportunity to experience our own way of thinking by hearing or reading what we have to say.

The inner ability to communicate enables us to formulate thoughts and share those with others. The action of thinking related to the Throat Chakra is a process of identifying and organizing consciousness for the purpose of transmitting consciousness. Communication organizes and expands thinking. When preparing for a lecture, the lecturer unites consciousness around a central idea. In the communication of this idea there is a time of shared consciousness between the lecturer and his audience. In this way, man is able to extend beyond the limitations of his own physical body which would otherwise cause him to be isolated from his environment.

Communication provides mobility. Physical mobility occurs through the movement of the physical body. Mentally, it occurs through projected thought. The Throat Chakra is the meeting point for energies used to produce abstract ideals which will eventually become a part of our manifested world. The will becomes the conveyor to transmit consciousness in order to cause a difference in our Selves and our world. Through the sharing of ideas and concepts of how we individually see the world we are able to influence those around us. This is why teaching is valued. Teaching is perhaps the highest form of expression available to man.

Communication can take many forms. The artist creates and arranges visual images with a particular thought in mind. Those who view his work will receive his idea in direct proportion to the artist's knowledge and skill in using the medium in ways that are easily identifiable. When abstract, the images hold meaning only for the artist and his message is lost. The viewer's mind is stimulated by what he sees, and he is free to invent his own interpretation of the artwork. Either way, communication has occurred.

Communication is often visual, but it can also be auditory, kinesthetic, dramatic, or literary. Any of the art forms serve man as a vehicle for Self expression. When viewed as a society, the arts provide culture which gives meaning to a group of individuals. There is creative artistry in any form of Self expression. Adornment of the physical body is a daily means of Self expression. From the way we style our hair to the color and texture of the clothing we wear, we make a personal statement about who we are in the appearance we present to others.

Today, electronic media is the most widely available avenue for global communication. Media exposes the mind of humanity to common experience. Whether discoveries or disasters, information is disseminated across miles of physical separation in a matter of hours. This access to communication makes the world seem a smaller place to live for it empowers us with the simultaneous viewing of events. The shared experience produces a group consciousness of how we perceive our world. It brings to us the opportunity to experience through someone else's eyes, and holds the potential for the acceleration of our evolution as humanity.

Electronic media has altered our concepts of time and space. Communication which a century ago took months to occur between sender and receiver, can now be enjoyed in a matter of minutes. Electronic media has given us the power of communication at will. This changes how we see our Selves and others. It stretches the imagination past self-imposed limits, demanding that man's ability to reason be accelerated. It is only through reasoning that we can separate fact from fiction, reality from fantasy, and the importance of this has never been greater than it is today primarily due to mass communication.

Each of the senses are vehicles for Self expression. It is sound that primarily manifests itself through the Throat Chakra energies. A mantra is a repetition of a sound or vibration. It is a word or group of words incorporating a musical tone. The verses of many familiar songs are mantras, so are many religious prayers. The word mantra is from the Sanskrit *man* meaning mind and *tra* meaning projection or instrument. How sounds are used affect how well we receive communicated messages. The choice of words to describe our thoughts can either create a rapport with the listener or repulse him. As a means of Self expression for the inattentive, the words we choose to convey our thoughts will convey much more than ideas. They will tell the listener who we are as well as what we think.

The vibrational patterns used in sound focus thoughts in a particular direction. Sounds have the meaning ascribed to them because of the rhythm they produce. Vowels are receptive and consonants are aggressive. The flowing rhythm of Latin or French have earned these languages the descriptive receptive title of romance languages while the guttural sounds of German are definitely aggressive. Vibrational patterns can also be identified in the difference between a classical music piece and jazz, rap music and a lullaby.

Moving up the ladder of the chakra system, we reach the point where we are able to choose to create the experiences that will enhance understanding of Self as a creator. We realize the wealth of opportunity for learning can only be useful as wise choices are made. By successively determining the quality and direction of our creative endeavors we define our unique form of expression. This expression requires not only the inner communication necessary for creative endeavor, but outer communication as well. Remember, communication is dual. It is both given and received. To utilize this chakra's energy strive to receive communication as well as offer it for it is the refined quality of receiving that will heighten and expand the quality of what you give.

In Sanskrit, this chakra is known as *Vissudha* meaning purification. The exactness with which we communicate creates a pure vision of how we perceive our world. For accurate communication to be given and received, the thoughts and verbal description of those thoughts need to be aligned. Otherwise, the receiver notes inconsistencies or untruths in what is being presented.

The Throat Chakra is typically illustrated with sixteen petals. Numerologically, sixteen digits to a seven, the number signifying direction or control. In the Buddhist tradition there are seven heavens. The Chinese recognize seven stars of the Great Bear in connection with seven bodily openings and seven openings of the human heart. In the mythology of Greece, seven was sacred to Apollo, the sun God. We also find seven gates of Thebes, seven sons of Helios, seven sons and seven daughters of Niobe, and seven wise men. In the Bible the number seven appears often in the book of *Revelation,* seven seals on the scroll, seven heavens of angelic hosts, seven heads on the beast, and seven cups of divine wrath. The most magnificent collection of architectural structures, the wonders of the ancient world, also number seven.

The most productive use of the Throat Chakra energies comes when the thoughts and words are aligned in communication. By developing listening skills, our ability to receive communication is enhanced. Being able to still the mind for reception is an art developed through practice. Stilling the mind frees the listener to receive complete communication from the mental as well as the physical senses. This enables the listener to develop the science of telepathy necessary for complete communication to occur.

Love used in communication is the key to the charismatic quality and is the result of the building process of becoming a creator. As the mind is awakened to the beauty of the creative process, the independent movement of the receptive and aggressive qualities unite and merge to produce the desired insight. This process is love in motion. It is expansive by nature and attracting through its order. Thus when communication is the result of a greater inner knowledge of the qualities of creation, the communicator has awareness of both his own need to give and the listener's need to receive. Charisma occurs when the communicator has the ability to give and receive at will.

The Throat Chakra will seem to move brighter and faster in public speakers and singers for they draw upon and utilize this energy continually. How charismatic they are will depend upon their ability to make quick decisions based upon not only what they desire to give but equally upon what they are receiving from their audience. This adeptness in including the audience in their decisions empowers the speaker or singer with the inner secrets of the Throat Chakra energy. With the complete use of this center, we find the full expression of creativity and an obvious personal integrity becomes evident in our expression of Self. By using this chakra's energies we realize the power of volition, the right to determine the quality and kind of thoughts we will express and receive, is in our hands.

Falling into habitual communication is one of the most widespread misuses of this center. When very little thought is given to what is said, communication is stymied. This mental laziness promotes stagnation in the minds of speaker and listener. Communication becomes disorganized, haphazard, incomplete, and worthless. The individual finds himself saying, "that's not what I meant" or "you know" as if he expected the listener to think and express for him. The listener finds himself asking, "What did you say?" for his attention has wandered and he has lost track of the speaker's message. Scattering of the attention will also cause a failure of accurately describing what is in the mind. When continued over a period of time, the misuse of energy will eventually affect the operation of the thyroid gland in the body.

Refusing to say what is on your mind, as if something is "caught in your throat", will produce laryngitis or tonsillitis. The virus which precipitates the common cold is usually present in the body. For it to take root, the thinker must be experiencing prolonged indecision. Indecisiveness directly limits Self expression, retarding Throat Chakra energies, thus leaving an open and susceptible place for the virus to become active.

To stimulate the action of the Thoat Chakra, first, teach. If you have children respect your position as teacher. You are entrusted with young minds. Teach the purpose and value of actions. Teach adults. You have people around you who admire your abilities. Teach them what you know about swimming, singing, salesmanship, parenting, cooking, experimenting. Second, become descriptive. Read descriptive passages in novels. Read poetry, becoming familiar with imagery. Practice describing physical objects while someone else draws what you describe. Third, practice listening. Learn to still the mind so you can receive a complete impression in your consciousness.

The Brow Chakra

Instinctually, the Brow Chakra is the *chakra of insight*. The quality of thinking governing its action can be termed Self Integration. How completely we know our Selves and our world depends on our willingness to perceive. To accurately evaluate the Self, we must be physically observant of the world around us. This observation occurs not only through the visual sense, but through the use of all senses. As the attention unites what is received from the physical senses, Spiritual perception is born. Spiritual perception transcends physical limitations of space and time. With the skill of perception we can separate and blend any idea, molding it to meet our creative specifications.

Often described as the "Third Eye", the Brow Chakra energies work directly with the master gland of the physical body, the pituitary gland. Located very close to the center of the brain, the third eye aptly describes this gland. The third eye symbolically represents the well developed and attuned use of what is termed the sixth sense. Attention is the only sense the mind has. When used in conjunction with the working of the five physical senses, attention opens the realms of mental perception. Most people never realize the power of Self because they are constantly scattering their attention and wasting mental energy. By learning to focus your attention on a single point at will, you become a master of your mental sense and prepare the mind for expansion.

Concentrative power is most easily developed by the highly intelligent and talented mind and is a prominent characteristic of genius. For this reason a practice of concentration is a prerequisite for Kundalini arousal. The aim of concentration is to attain one-pointedness of mind by keeping only one object or line of thought before the mind. When practicing concentration, you must stay alert, not allowing the mind to drift into unconsciousness. This is the difference between a passive, inwardly focused mental condition and the alert, attentive and controlled focused state. Disciplining the mind continues until the mind becomes accustomed to holding any desired image. When this is achieved we are free to experience mental perception.

With mental perception we can realize the separation of the inner Self and the outer Self. We discriminate between the parts of Self directly related to the physical world and the parts of Self existing beyond the physical, those belonging to the spiritual world. This becomes known through the development of the power of reasoning and the power of intuition. When the mind is directed toward the creation of an ideal and purpose, there is the freedom to begin building reasoning. When memory, attention, and imagination are effectively combined, we find the benefit of reasoning is the production of intuition. Intuition is the direct grasp of Truth.

Use of the Brow Chakra energies is a result of familiarity with the five lower chakras. Since these energies respond to active mental direction only, you will want to provide your Self with a strong Spiritual foundation. This is built through the development of the quality of thinking governing the lower chakra centers. Awaken your consciousness by pursuing Self Autonomy, Self Reliance, Self Identity, Self Acceptance, and Self Awareness. To be free to integrate consciousness means you have identified the parts of Self that will form the whole.

Utilizing the flow of the Brow Chakra energies, heightens the individual's intuitive or psychic perceptions. Reasoning gives us the power to create the fulfillment of consciously produced desires. By utilizing Brow Chakra energies we open our Selves to the fulfillment of desires beyond the physical.

What is permanent becomes paramount. We realize what we need to know and understand is creation. Thus how we know Self as a creator becomes the motivation for the integration of Self.

Now the past, present, and future can be effectively used to produce not only the kind of life we want but the kind of being we desire. Intuition gives us the power to expand and accelerate the fulfillment of desires. One use of intuition is the perception of lines of probabilities. Here the past, present, and future are perceived to elevate awareness beyond physical limitations. With developed intuition we can identify how today relates to previous lifetimes, we can determine the timing of the manifestation of desires, and we can develop the skill of prophecy. Understandings we have previously gained also become apparent. Once consciously acknowledged, these understandings from the past can be called into action in the present to accelerate our growth and development.

The Sanskrit word for this chakra is *Ajna* meaning to perceive or to command. It is sometimes called Shiva Netra, Shiva's Eye, or the eye of wisdom. The petals of this chakra are illustrated as 96 which digits to a six. Six is the number of service. Those who use this chakra's energies will always be found in service endeavors. They are the people who have a career not just a job. Their minds are consistently active toward the betterment of Self and others. They live with a constant awareness that how they think is just as important as what they think. They experience an inner drive toward completion (as symbolized by the "9") whether it comes in the form of Self integration or the integration of mankind. In time, these awarenesses grow into the realization and fulfillment of man's destiny to become a spiritual being.

This chakra is dual in nature and illustrations show it as being divided into halves among the many petals. This duality represents the manifested and the unmanifested. This is the point where the ida and pingala meet. This duality is symbolized by the number two. Pythagoras noted that the number two was the first true number because it represented the first plurality.

Two gives birth to multiplicity. It is symbolic of doubling, separation, and opposition. The dualism can be seen throughout the mythology of the world in the creator and the created, light and shadow, male and female, spirit and matter, good and evil, life and death, right and left, yin and yang. The principles of good *(Ahura Mazda)* and evil *(Ahriman)* formed the basis of Zarathustra's teachings.

The productive use of this chakra's energy results in direct perception. The effective use of the past by drawing upon memory and of the future through the imagination, expands consciousness and leads to a fulfilling and progressive life. The individual who can immediately identify cause and cure when a problem arises is drawing upon this center's energy. By understanding that thought is cause and the physical is its manifest likeness we heighten our perception of existence. We are free to perceive on more than one level of awareness. We understand that a broken arm has a physical cause which is abnormal stress to the bone, a mental cause of inattentiveness which produced the physical stress, and a spiritual cause resulting in the susceptibility of the weakened bone structure. This multi-dimensional perception enhances the full spectrum of creativity. Inventiveness finds its greatest expression through the use of the Brow Chakra.

Effectively balancing daydreams and night dreams results in full use of the Brow Chakra energies. Clairvoyant experiences are common. Beyond unwanted and uncontrolled visions, the individual who uses these energies does so with awareness and direction. Visions or precognitive dreams are no longer seen as a warning of possible danger. They are perceived as an impetus for the further development of mankind requiring cultivation and employment to manifest their destiny.

With this center the seat of divine intelligence becomes known, and we find new realities for Self manifesting in the physical plane. We leave behind comparisons of Self based upon what has been done before or what the majority are presently doing. Through Self evaluation we truly begin to lead our own life according to the highest principles we can perceive.

Life becomes a series of choices of what to do and for what purpose, rather than a series of forced changes made from what we want to avoid experiencing.

Misuse of the Brow Chakra energies are the result of confusing the past, present, and future. When someone physically ages, but endeavors to remain the same he begins forfeiting the learning of today and in his mind he lives in the past. This can manifest as physical imbalance resulting in Alzheimer's disease. Repeatedly refusing to utilize reasoning will manifest in nervous system disorders. A nervous breakdown is the result of consciously avoiding experiences in the life. Wanting to shut out stimuli from the outer environment as received through the senses will cause pituitary disorders. Wanting to shut out stimuli from the inner environment leads to paranoia or schizophrenia. All difficulties related to the misuse of Brow Chakra energies arise from some type of refusal to use the life for learning.

To stimulate the Brow Chakra energies, first, give your Self a daily IQ test. This is your intuitive quotient. Begin describing your intuitive experiences on paper. The precognitive dream you had, the parking space you expected and received, or knowing who was on the other end of the telephone are examples of experiences you will want to record. Second, practice undivided attention. Set aside a ten minute period of time daily for focusing your attention upon a single object. Use the same object each day. Cause your mind to remain focused upon that object during the time allotted. Fill your mind in one-pointed concentration only. Be persistent. Your mind is yours to use. Train it to do what you desire then you can use it for transcendent pursuits.

The Crown Chakra

The Crown Chakra is instinctually the *chakra of fulfill-ment*. The quality of thinking governing its action can be termed Self Transcendence. Here duality is transcended and the individual experiences wholeness. Integration has been achieved and the attention is now directed toward the inner worlds releasing the physical experiences which produced this understanding. Creation is now in harmony and we find the release of attachment through fulfillment to become a real probability in our lives. The singular awareness of the self transcended is that learning is the only desire remaining to be fulfilled.

There is a wonderful parable illustrating the thoughts of one who uses this chakra. There was a man who had more riches than he could use. He was content with his life except he repeatedly experienced debilitations of his physical body. The illnesses increased with age. He often found himself with the money to do whatever he wanted, but his weakened body did not allow him to spend it in ways he desired.

When the man was nearing death he inwardly prayed to his maker, "If I am to born again, I shall be a happy man if you will give me a strong, healthy body. I will not care if I have riches or not. Just let me be healthy."

When he reincarned, he was born into a poor family. He had a strong body, but found it increasingly difficult due to his poverty to provide his body with the necessary sustenance it required. When he neared death from starvation, he prayed, "I have a strong body but what good is it without the money to buy food? If I must be born again, please give me money and health and I will be happy."

In his third incarnation, the man found himself incarned as a woman. She was healthy and wealthy but rather plain looking and lacked the charm needed to be attractive to the opposite sex. As she aged, she found her life unsatisfying for lack of someone to share her good fortune. So when the woman was dying she prayed, "If I must be born again, please do not let me be lonely. I will be happy if I have health, wealth, beauty, and the gift of conversation so I may find someone who will share my life."

In her fourth incarnation, the woman found herself wealthy, healthy, and beautiful. She expressed herself with ease and in time she met and married a handsome man. After several years, her husband died unexpectedly and she spent the remainder of her years in mourning. When she approached death, with a broken heart she prayed, "If I am to be born again, in addition to health, wealth, and attractiveness, please bring me a mate who will live long and share my joy."

In her fifth incarnation, the woman found herself again in a male body. He enjoyed the fulfillment of all his desires including the mate he had wanted. In time, his wife's beauty faded and as she took him for granted she became more and more critical with each passing day making his life miserable. When he approached death he prayed, "You have given me all I requested. If I am to be born again, could you please send me a wife who will be more positive and appreciative?"

In his sixth incarnation, the man enjoyed the fulfillment of all his desires. In time he even met and married a wonderful woman who attended to his every need. He tired of her constant affection and his attention began to wander to other attractive females. Falling in love with a younger woman, he divorced his good wife and married his new love. In time, she left him for a younger man.

Distraught by this chain of events, the man prayed to his maker, "Lord you have given me everything I requested. You have given me many chances to be happy in life and each time there is something missing." His maker replied, "What would you ask of me now?" The man, wiser from his varied experiences, thought for a moment and responded, "I have sought happiness in many ways, only to find them bringing temporary joy. What I desire most of all is to have a happiness that lasts. Now, I realize all I want is constant awareness of you."

This story illustrates the progression of consciousness of one individual. It embodies the awakening to spiritual consciousness described in many of the world's myths. In the Bible, it was Solomon who realized he only wanted to know his Lord, and as a result was given the fulfillment of every desire. When consciousness has awakened to inner desire, we find all our needs are fulfilled and our outer desires are few. What previously kept us attached to physical people, places, and things, no longer attracts our attention for these have been utilized and understanding of their value has been made a part of Self. The lower consciousness has fulfilled its purpose for existence and now the consciousness reaches for awareness of the superconscious Self.

The individual who is prepared to use the Crown chakra energies finds the awareness of all - the omnipresent, the omnipotent, and the omniscient. This awareness has been described as the Buddha consciousness, the Christ consciousness, and the Cosmic consciousness. It is consciousness of the highest manifestation of Self as a creator. Such an individual is fully prepared to stimulate the use of Kundalini for he has come to understand the meaning of meeting God face to face.

Having accomplished this actualized state of being, the individual is never the same. There is no returning to old patterns of limited thinking or old ways of experiencing in the world. There is only identification with forward motion toward maturing as a whole Self. The inner urge toward enlightenment fills every thought seeking complete expression. The meaning of enlightenment is the ability to use all levels of consciousness simultaneously.

In the Sanskrit, this chakra is termed *Sahasara* meaning "thousandfold". This represents the one unity with the power produced from understanding. It is the God number, representing your true individuality. It is the totality into which all things and beings strive to mature.

The productive use of the Crown Chakra energies results in higher consciousness, the perception of a higher order. A sense of wholeness and transcendence of any limitation becomes part of the thoughts. There is an awareness of Self existing in an unchanging eternal present and a constant awareness of connection with the universe. There is no death when this state of consciousness is achieved for the illusion of separateness has been transcended.

Misuse of this energy occurs when the attention becomes mired in the limitations of the physical. Sensory attachment produces identification with the finite world grossly limiting the potential of Self. This causes a forfeiting of the creative ability of Self. Evolution is stymied and the energies remain stagnant. Prolonged identification with the physical results in deterioration of the functions of the body. Resiliency is lost, rejuvenation powers slowed, and disease appears in areas of the body most susceptible. Eventually there is physical death.

To stimulate the action of the Crown Chakra, first, prepare your body through physical disciplines. These include controlling the breath and heartbeat, inducing relaxation of muscles, and directing energy flows. Second, prepare the mind by fulfilling your desires. To release attachment to the physical, you must fulfill physical desires. Contemplate why people, places, and things in life are important to you. Seek the essence that gives meaning to your existence. Third, pray and meditate. Develop communion with your Creator.

By becoming familiar with the quality of thinking governing each chakra's action you can more easily identify your strengths and weaknesses. If you find Self Acceptance to be difficult, use your understanding of Self Reliance to foster purposefulness which will lead to Self Approval. By using the strength of one area of thinking you can build strength in another. When all characteristics described are developed, the Self becomes unified functioning as a whole and healthy being. This expanded awareness prepares you for the use of the greatest creative energy known to man - the Kundalini.

And yes, there are two chakras which function beyond the vibratory creation of mind. These are present in reasoning man but rarely used. As consciousness expands causing man's next evolutionary step into Spiritual Man these centers will become more prominent. They can be perceived by one who has awakened the Kundalini and directs her at will.

The first is what can be termed the I Am Chakra. This is the fully awakened consciousness, the mature sense of *I* experienced outwardly in the ego chakra. This awakening corresponds to union of two Eastern dieties known as Shakti, the feminine principle, and Shiva, the masculine principle. Shiva symbolizes the male. He is formless, the inactivated divine potential, the existence of pure consciousness. Shiva pushes out from above through the irresistible attraction of divine grace or manifestation. Shakti symbolizes the female. She is the life giver, the substance of a manifested universe. She is the projection of consciousness. The root word of Shakti is *Shak* meaning to have power or to be able. Signifying receptivity, Shakti produces a universe only with the seed of consciousness from Shiva. Shakti pulls up from earth the divine aspiration of the human soul and the individual knows who he is as a matured offspring of his maker.

The final chakra center is the Light Chakra. These are the energies of the alpha and omega. Here is experienced Saraswati and Brahman, the duality of God made whole by awareness. The mother being feminine and receptive is existence. The father being masculine and aggressive is free will. Both are the essence of primal creativity, the creativity which sparks the birth of a new universe.

This is the epitome of creativity. By transcending one's Self, creation is known. What lies beyond transcendence is found in the sacred knowledge of Kundalini.

The Chakras in Spiritual Literature

The conscious and intentional use of Kundalini requires knowledge of the Self beyond the physical. Kundalini is the most powerful of all energies available to man because it is the energy of Spirit. By becoming familiar with the mental energies transformed by the major chakras, you prepare your mind and heart for the raising of the Kundalini.

The chakras are much more than etheric devices which keep the body healthy. Since they recycle energies in the inner levels of consciousness, chakras assist in the balancing of energy and serve the very important function of replenishing the inner Self's energy supply. In addition to the expansion of consciousness that comes with proper chakra function, knowing how to direct the chakra functions is a prerequisite to raising the Kundalini because you will need to know how to stimulate your chakras into action following the energy use occurring during the raising of Kundalini.

We have discussed the chakras and their function in detail. Now it is time to explore the origin and development of the chakra system. Cosmic energy pervades the universe. It energizes your consciousness through the awareness of your being as an individual. From that point of reception it energizes your mind beginning in the superconscious mind and feeding the subconscious mind, and finally the conscious mind. When cosmic energy enters the physical body through the medulla oblongota it becomes the life force for your physical body. How the reception of cosmic energy was created is described in the spiritual literature of the world.

Exploring inner ecology is part of the intent behind the world's mythological stories and Holy scriptures. The scriptures of the world endeavor to explain the principles of creation through parables and myths. Each describe man's experience in and relationship to his universe through the use of allegories. This enables the listener or reader to interpret the stories according to his or her understanding. Man is dual in nature, both inner and outer, spiritual and material. When we study these stories with an eye to the universality of the tale we begin to use the wisdom of the ages to understand our existence of today.

In Hindu teachings the nature of energy is described by the triune gods, Brahma, Vishnu, and Siva. Brahma represents and creates energy. Brahma is pictured with four heads and four hands. He had five heads until Siva cut one off. He is paired with Saraswati the goddess of poetry, wisdom and eloquence who is the daughter of Kama, the god of love.

Vishnu preserves energy. He has four hands and is paired with his wife Lakshmi the goddess of wealth and beauty.

Siva destroys energy. He has four hands and three eyes. One of the eyes has the power to kill. He lives in the Himalayas and is known as the Lord of the Mountain. He is the god of arts and knowledge. His wife Bhanani aids him by using a rope to strangle the wicked.

Vishnu sleeps on Ananta, the serpent that lives forever. At the end of the present age of the world, the Kali Yuga as it is known, a lotus will grow from his navel. The waters of the world will cover everything and on the lotus Brahma will appear to again carry out his periodic task of creating the earth anew.

These vivid images convey the constant motion characteristic of cosmic energy. By bringing together the god and goddess, the aggressive and receptive principles can work together to produce creation. Brahma represents creative material, energy in its unformed state. Siva represents the transformation of energy from one form to another, always in alignment with what will produce progression. Vishnu represents the creative potential of awakened Kundalini.

How man uses this cosmic energy as his own life force is described in the Bible. Early Biblical stories refer to a river rising up in Eden to water the garden where the newly created man exists. This river divides into four branches. Symbolically this describes the reception of cosmic energy into the physical body where it becomes the individual's life force. Students of metaphysics learn how to control this cosmic energy. They practice drawing cosmic energy into the physical body through focused mental direction. This is learned through developing healing abilities, by directing the action of the major-minor and minor chakras of the body, and by developing control of the Kundalini energy.

Important to one who desires to use Kundalini is the knowledge of what causes the mind to be energized. This myth reveals when man was formed he became a living being because the Lord God breathed the breath of life into him. In an earlier chapter we discussed the duty of the superconscious mind. This duty is to supply energy to the rest of mind. Without a supplier of energy within your own consciousness, you would not exist as a physical being or as a thinker. Two physical adults can come together to produce an offspring, but unless there is a soul willing to inhabit the created vehicle, once separated from the mother the "child" will not live. There must be a part of mind responsible for supplying energy from the innermost part of you to the outermost and that is the duty of your superconscious mind. Through the soul, the subconscious mind receives this energy and in turn energizes the conscious mind, thus producing a living being functioning independently of its parents.

When Kundalini awakens, she leaves revelation in her path. The most specific writings in spiritual literature describing the experience of Kundalini appear in the last book in the Bible: *Revelation*. In fact, the development of Kundalini can be traced throughout these scriptures. In the story of Cain, we find a symbolic representation of the creation of the major chakra centers. Cain is the first offspring of Adam and Eve, who represent the formation of the subconscious and conscious minds respectively. Cain was a tiller of the soil. Adam and Eve also produced another son named Abel who was a keeper of the flocks. Both brothers created offerings for the Lord God. Abel's gift was looked upon favorably while Cain's wasn't. Cain was crestfallen because of this. When Cain and Abel were out in the field, Cain decided to slay his brother, thinking he could get away with it. As we learn very quickly when you study Biblical myths, the Lord God knows what is going on, when it is going on, and usually before it goes on. The Lord God symbolizes the inner urge to be compatible to our maker and thus displays omniscient perception. The Lord asks Cain where his brother is. Even if you are not a Biblical scholar, you're probably familiar with Cain's response, *"Am I my brother's keeper?"* The Lord knows what Cain has done and he curses Cain. He tells Cain he will no longer be a tiller of the soil. From this time forward he will be a restless wanderer. Cain responds that his punishment is too great to bear. He realizes he is being sent away from the presence of the Lord and he believes anyone will be able to kill him at sight. The Lord receives this and responds saying no. "If anyone slays Cain, Cain will be avenged sevenfold."

This story describes a development in man's evolution which occurred thousands of years ago. As cosmic energy enters man to become his life force, the need arises for man to be responsible for that energy. In taking responsibility for using this energy, man also accepts responsibility for replenishing it. By recycling energy that he has used, man can insure his continued existence. The "mark of Cain" represents taking on that responsibility of learning in the physical existence. The physical will be where we as thinkers can learn and progress spiritually. The energies we use will be manifested in the physical plane of existence, *"away from the presence of the Lord"*. This will be accomplished through the establishment of seven energy transformers or what we have referred to as chakras.

There was a point in time in your evolution when you *"killed Abel"* which is why you have been avenged sevenfold. When you and I killed *"Abel"* the physical became our only place to learn through this stage of our evolution.

Between Cain and the next Biblical parable concerning the use of the chakras there were several individuals whose names you will probably recognize. There was a series of covenants between these people and the Lord God. The first was a man named Abram who became Abraham once the covenant was established. His son Isaac, and his son Jacob, represent steps in the development of the thinker. These three illustrate significant developments in how the conscious mind, the subconscious mind, and the superconscious mind will be used to promote evolutionary progression.

There is a story often called Jacob's ladder which describes the chakra system. At Bethel, Jacob falls asleep and has a dream. The dream is of a stairway that rests on the ground and its top reaches all the way to heaven. God's messengers or angels move up and down this stairway. The Lord is standing beside Jacob and says, *"I the Lord am the God of your forefather Abraham and the God of Isaac. The land upon which you are lying I will give to you and your descendents. These shall be as plentiful as the dust of the earth and through them you shall spread out east and west and north and south. In you and your descendants all the nations of the earth shall find blessing. Know that I Am with you. I will protect you wherever you go and bring you back to this land. I will never leave you until I have done what I have promised you."* (Genesis 28:13-15) Jacob's dream is similar to the mystical experience of the spontaneous arousal of Kundalini. He receives his vision or mission through a dream. The *stairway* is the chakra system and the *angels* are the qualities of thinking governing each chakra. These are to be used for spiritual development by replenishing the mind's *earth* or substance with the energy needed for creation.

A little later in the account of Jacob's life, he struggles with a man until the break of day. As a result of that experience Jacob's name is changed to *Israel* and he realizes he has contended with divine and human beings and his life has been spared. He also realizes that he has met God face to face. This awareness is alive in anyone who knows he exists beyond the physical. By confronting and accepting the Spiritual essence of Self, we are free to respond to both outer and inner stimuli. When you know how to control the chakras and the highest energies that are available to man, this is an experience of *meeting God face to face* because you realize your own divinity.

Jacob's stairway experience and the Lord God's promise reveal the purpose for our responsibility of returning the energy we have used in creating back into the inner levels of mind. This purpose is to become compatible to the Creator who brought us into existence. Until this point in evolution as it is described in the Bible, we were only responsible for our learning in the physical plane. Because of the changes in consciousness which have occurred symbolized in the passages from Cain to Jacob, we now have a glimpse of a greater purpose for possessing these seven major energy transformers.

The next major Biblical reference to the chakras occurs with Moses in the book of *Exodus*. Moses symbolically represents the development and use of the imagination. You are probably familiar with Moses as being the one who led the Israelites during a time they were in bondage in Egypt under Pharaoh. With the help of the Lord, Moses stimulated Pharaoh through a variety of plagues to let the Israelites go. You might also remember Moses because he was the one who received the ten commandments from the Lord.

There was something else that Moses did. With his aid Joshua, Moses went to a mountain after having received the ten commandments. This time he was instructed by the Lord to build a sanctuary so the Lord could dwell in the Israelites' midst. The 25th chapter of *Exodus* gives a detailed account of what Moses is to build. This becomes known as the ark of the covenant. The materials that will be used to build this ark, the way it will be fashioned, and what will be placed in it including the ten commandments are described in detail. Beginning with verse 31, the Lord instructs Moses on the building of the lampstand: *"You shall make a lampstand of pure beaten gold, its shaft and branches, with its cups and knobs and petals springing directly from it. Six branches are to extend from the sides of the lampstand, three branches on one side, and three on the other. On one branch there are to be three cups, shaped like almond blossoms, each with its knob and petals; on the opposite branch there are to be three cups, shaped like almond blossoms, each with its knob and petals; and so for the six branches that extend from the lampstand. On the shaft there are to be four cups, shaped like almond blossoms, with their knobs and petals, including a knob below each of the three pairs of branches that extend from the lampstand. Their knobs and branches shall so spring from it that the whole will form but a single piece of pure beaten gold. You shall then make seven lamps for it and so set up the lamps that they shed their light on the space in front of the lampstand. These, as well as the trimming shears and trays, must be of pure gold. Use a talent of pure gold for the lampstand and all its appurtenances. See that you make them according to the pattern shown you on the mountain." (Exodus 25:31-40)*

The key to this is *"their knobs and branches shall so spring from it that the whole will form but a single piece of pure beaten gold"*. There is a relationship that each of the major chakras have with one another. There is no one chakra that stands independently of the others. Each chakra recycles energy back into mind not in a linear fashion but in an inclusive fashion. Each chakra will return energy into more than one level of consciousness. This inclusion of several levels will be explained later in passages from the book of *Revelation*.

The instructions for building the ark of the covenant symbolize another step that has been taken in the development of the chakras. This step is the interrelationship of all the chakras. They will all work together to produce a whole, functioning Self or an I Am with awareness. The chakra system will be singular in its ideal and purpose even while comprised of seven individual pieces.

Joshua's story also lends insight into the development of the chakras. When Moses died, Joshua succeeded him. Joshua leads the Israelites across the Jordan River and they bring the ark of the covenant with them. Once the ark is made it goes everywhere with the Israelites. The Lord promised he would deliver to Joshua and the Israelites a city called Jericho. Jericho is the oldest known city in the world. The Lord told Joshua I'm going to let you take this city, but this is what you've got to do. For six days, the soldiers have to march around the city. The priests will carry ram's horns and the ark of the covenant marching with the soldiers. On the seventh day, they will march around the city seven times. After this seventh time, the priests will blow their horns and the people will shout, and this is how the Lord will deliver the city.

All upright and righteous men listen to the Lord, so Joshua does what the Lord says. At the end of the seventh circling of the city, the horns are blown, the people shout, and the walls of the city crumble. That enables Joshua and the Israelites to storm into the city and kill every living creature by sword. Joshua then places a curse. His oath before the Lord is that any man who attempts to rebuild this city will lose his first born when the foundation is laid and lose his youngest when the gates are made.

The place that this story symbolically holds in the development for us as thinkers and the use of the chakras is to be able to go beyond any limitations that might exist toward this purpose of becoming a creator which has already been established in order to achieve awareness. We find throughout the Bible, from this time forward, anytime there is the sounding of trumpets or horns they signify a use of the chakra energies.

Some time passes between Joshua and the next Biblical character we will discuss. David was a shepherd boy who became a king. He had been king for quite a while, so long that he had a moment of respite from fighting. David had many enemies and fought for most of his life. This story occurs at a point when he is at rest from his enemies. He says to Nathan, the prophet who aided David, here I am living in a house of cedar while the ark of God dwells in a tent. Perhaps he was thinking, God really should have something better than a tent. Nathan, who was his advisor, told him okay, go ahead and do whatever you want to do and the Lord will be with you. The Lord, however, has something else in mind. The story is described this way: *"But that night the Lord spoke to Nathan and said, 'Go, tell my servant David, Thus says the Lord: Should you build me a house to dwell in? I have not dwelt in a house from the day on which I led the Israelites out of Egypt to the present, but I have been going about in a tent under cloth. In all my wanderings everywhere among the Israelites, did I ever utter a word to any one of the judges whom I charged to tend my people Israel, to ask: Why have you not built me a house of cedar?' Now then, speak thus to my servant David, 'The Lord of hosts has this to say: It was I who took you from the pasture and from the care of the flock to be commander of my people Israel. I have been with you wherever you went, and I have destroyed all your enemies before you. And I will make you famous like the great ones of the earth. I will fix a place for my people Israel; I will plant them so that they may dwell in their place without further disturbance. Neither shall the wicked continue to afflict them as they did of old, since the time I first appointed judges over my people Israel. I will give you rest from all your enemies. The Lord also reveals to you that he will establish a house for you. And when your time comes and you rest with your ancestors, I will raise up your heir after you, sprung from your loins, and I will make his kingdom firm. It is he who shall build a house for my name. And I will make his royal throne firm forever. I will be a father to him, and he shall be a son to me. And if he does wrong, I will correct him with the rod of men and with human chastisements; but I will not withdraw my favor from him as I withdrew it from your predecessor Saul, whom I removed from my presence. Your house and your kingdom shall endure forever before me; your throne shall stand firm forever.' Nathan reported all these words and this entire vision to David."* (II Samuel 7:8-17)

When you study the life of David you realize he signifies the development of reasoning. It is not that David knew how to reason, but rather through his actions he learned what it takes to be able to reason. His life incorporates memory, attention, and imagination. The stories of his life illustrate the discovery of these elements and how they can be coordinated to produce reasoning. David wanted very much to build the house he never got to build, that was the duty of his son, Solomon. Experimentation and experience through reasoning alone is incomplete for reaching the state of transcendence. David did not have everything required to cause the change. It requires the understanding and wisdom symbolized by Solomon to cause the next stage of evolution of the soul. Understanding the quality of thinking governing each chakra needs to become part of the Self to pave the way for the Kundalini to become active.

When we reach Jesus and the New Testament of the Bible, we find a further use of the chakras as illustrated in the story of the fishes and loaves. The story is set in Bethsaida where Jesus is teaching. His apostles come to him asking him to let the people go so they can find lodging and food. Jesus looks at his disciples and says why don't you feed them? The apostles reply there are five thousand men to feed and they only have five loaves and two fishes. Jesus thinks about that and says to divide the crowd into groups of fifty. The apostles respond. Jesus takes the five loaves and two fishes and blesses them. He then hands these to the apostles who distribute it to this group of five thousand men. After everyone has eaten everything they can handle there is still enough to fill twelve baskets. Now, how did he do that?

The five loaves are symbolic of the five lower chakras. These are the chakras that directly affect and work with the reenergizing of your conscious and subconscious minds. The two fishes are symbolic of the two higher chakras that work with the recycling of energy into the superconscious mind. The twelve apostles represent the twelve major aspects of the conscious mind. Jesus is usually in control of the situations described during his life. This symbolizes the ability to give direction to the many aspects of Self. When there is one directing intelligence for the Self there is effective use of energy. Since Jesus represents the individual who is striving to know who he is and become Christ conscious, he represents you as an individual and how you can live now. You have within your power to use every ounce of energy fully, wasting nothing.

The parables of Jesus and his life describe how we are to live now as reasoning man. The *Book of Revelation* symbolically describes our destiny as Spiritual man. It instructs us on how to use reasoning man fully producing intuitive consciousness. Revelation is a book that has confounded people of all generations since the time it was written. It is very exciting for a metaphysician to study and put into practice the symbology of its instruction.

In the first chapter it speaks of seven lampstands of gold. We have already read of a lampstand of gold back in Exodus with the ark of the covenant. This is not the first lampstand of gold, but in the Revelation we have seven lampstands of gold. Among them is one like a son of man. Later in the chapter it tells us the secret meaning of the seven lampstands. It says the seven lampstands are the seven churches which sounds revealing but what are the seven churches?

When you read chapters two and three, you discover what these churches are. These churches describe the spiritual qualities and area of influence of each chakra. But decoding the symbology we discover how each chakra functions, why it functions as it does, and what we can produce when it functions properly. In describing each church, the Lord makes what sounds like accusations to the individual who is learning about these energy transformers.

The first church is Ephesus. During the passage on Ephesus, the Lord says *"you have turned away from your early love."* The early love we understand to be your subconscious mind. This means with this chakra you have turned all your attention to the physical, only thinking of fulfilling physical desires. This is the way you have been using your energy giving absolutely no thought to any kind of permanent understanding. No thought to heavenly treasures that you might take with you. No thought to how your soul could progress through the thoughts and actions you are taking.

Ephesus is symbolic of the thinking governing the root chakra. The quality of the root chakra is creativity. It symbolizes your ability to create, to be able to imagine something you desire and expect it to occur. This is in response to an inner urge, the urge to build.

The second church is Smyrna. Part of what the Lord says about Smyrna is that he is very much aware of your trials and tribulations and your poverty even though you are rich. Smyrna represents the thinking governing the adrenal chakra. The quality of this chakra is power but more important than that it is a response to an inner urge. The inner urge is for freedom.

The next church is Pergamum. The Lord says he knows that you live in the place where Satan's throne is erected. Pergamum represents the thinking governing the solar plexus chakra. The solar plexus is the seat of the conscious and subconscious minds. Its quality is balance. The balance it addresses is not whether you will do one thing or another in the physical; this balance is the full use of the conscious and subconscious minds as a unit. The solar plexus chakra exists in response to an inner urge. This inner urge is for direction.

The next church is Thyatira. The Lord says you tolerate a Jezebel that self-styled prophetess. The Lord also promises that the victor will receive the morning star. The morning star is Lucifer the most beautiful angel in heaven until he fell and became known as Satan. Thyatira represents the thinking governing the heart chakra. Thyatira's quality is understanding. It is in response to the inner urge for experiences to produce something permanent. By drawing upon what has been gained through productively using the earlier chakras will can produce understandings which will last.

The next church is Sardis. The Lord says, *"I know your reputation for being alive when in fact you are dead."* Here, the Lord also promises that the victor's name will go into the book of the living. The victor spoken of indicates the individual who has gained understanding of how to use these energy transformers. This understanding enables you to achieve a kind of victory. This victory is the control of your own mind.

Sardis represents the thinking governing the throat chakra. Its quality is choice. You may have heard it described as will, but choice more aptly conveys the idea of this chakra. Its inner urge is to cause motion or change. This completes the five lower chakras.

Next is the church in Philadelphia. Here the Lord speaks of *"an open door before you which no one can close"*. The victor in this case gains a pillar in the temple of God and experiences what is termed the New Jerusalem. Philadelphia represents the thinking governing the brow chakra. Its quality is reasoning, and it exists in response to the inner urge to discriminate.

Laodicea is the final church that is described in Revelation. The Lord says that *"you are neither hot nor cold, how I wish you were either hot or cold, but since you're lukewarm I will spew you out of my mouth"*. Later he says the victor, the one who learns about this chakra, will win the right to sit with me on my throne. Laodicea is the thinking governing the crown chakra, its quality is awareness, and it is in response to your inner urge to know the Christ consciousness.

Having studied the metaphysical truths in the Bible and Holy scriptures for years, I know the ideas I am sharing with you are true. I know that each individual who desires to know and is willing to fulfill that desire will discover these universal truths as they grow in their own truth.

The churches paint a picture of what is available right now for man to use. Some of its symbology may describe where you have come from, some will relate to where you are now in your awareness, and some conveys where this knowledge will lead you in the descriptions of the victories. However, it is not until later in *Revelation* that we find a symbolic description of the conscious experience of using chakra energies. If you desire, you can research this. You will want to find references to *trumpets* for they symbolize this activity. The imagery is rich with descriptions including hailstorms and a third of the earth being destroyed by locusts. But that is the subject of another book, The Universal Language of Mind: Book of Revelation Interpreted by Dr. Daniel R. Condron.

As you begin to build conscious control of the chakras you are climbing Jacob's ladder which was set into motion so long ago, you are feeding your five thousand, and your destiny becomes very clear. The eleventh chapter of Revelation gives us a clear image of this ideal for spiritual man in the description of the seventh trumpet. *"Then the seventh angel blew his trumpet. Loud voices in heaven cried out, 'The kingdom of the world now belongs to our Lord and to his Anointed One, and he shall reign forever and ever.' The twenty-four elders who were enthroned in God's presence fell down to worship God and said: 'We praise you, the Lord God Almighty, who is and who was. You have assumed your great power, you have begun your reign. The nations have raged in anger, but then came your day of wrath and the moment to judge the dead: The time to reward your servants the prophets and the holy ones who revere you, the great and the small alike; The time to destroy those who lay the earth waste.' Then God's temple in heaven opened and in the temple could be seen the ark of his covenant. There were flashes of lightning and peals of thunder, an earthquake, and a violent hailstorm."* This passage describes what occurs in the thinker when the energies of the crown chakra are consciously recognized. Light and sound are characteristic of the mystical experience produced by the spontaneous awakening of Kundalini.

By learning to direct the flow of the energies moving through your chakras, you show responsibility for your inner ecology. Your thinking is elevated toward the wise use of the creative energies available to you. You take greater care in what and how you create with developed precognition of how your creation will be useful. More and more you insure that any waste produced as a result of your creations can be used toward your next creation or be useful to other forms of creation. When you are inwardly responsible, it becomes a natural extension of your awareness to be outwardly responsible to your Self and humanity.

Learning to direct your chakra energies prepares you with the understanding necessary to use the Kundalini wisely. By using the serpent power man elevates his creativity beyond that of the creative genius and into the realms of his destiny as Spiritual Man.

A Serpent is Born

Once active, Kundalini produces transcendent states of awareness leading to enlightenment. She can also be used by the enlightened to transform substance. To wield her with awareness is to possess the power to transcend our dual nature creating wholeness of Self and communion with the creative forces of the universe. The reason for her existence is discovered in the parables of the world. By investigating these myths with an eye for what is universally applicable we become more acquainted with Kundalini, her nature and her relationship with man's consciousness.

Myths of transformation appear throughout the world's literature. Most often the serpent is used as a symbol for rebirth, regeneration, and change which leads to man's transformation from a thinking being entrapped in the physical senses into a thinker possessing the awareness of his reason for existence.

The myths of the world present the serpent or snake in a variety of forms and activities. How we regard the serpent depends upon the level of understanding we are willing to explore. The serpent can be merely another physical creature, a symbol of mental cunning, or an embodiment of spiritual evolution.

Physically, the snake represents a primary function of life - to eat. When we sit down to a meal most of us don't consider that what we're about to partake was very recently alive. This is true of flesh we eat, of meat, and it is also true of plant life. The less evolved life forms we use to sustain our physical bodies are living forces. The mythological snake represents a rejuvenation of life because in the physical there must be a killing in order for life to continue.

The serpent also represents the advantage of being born again. In the physical, you can very easily see this by observing the snake shedding its skin in order to be reborn. In many pictorial descriptions, the serpent is illustrated in a circle. The snake's mouth reaches until it is eating its own tail. This represents the image of life, the urge to be reborn, the never ending circle. One generation lends life to another generation. The old generation dies away and the new creates again. And this is the continuity of life which the serpent represents.

The serpent also represents an immortal energy in consciousness. It is constantly throwing off death and being reborn, so there is indeed everlasting life. Exploring myths can aid us to understand the symbolic relationship of the serpent to the Kundalini energy in man.

Although we tend to be afraid from our own ignorance of snakes in this country, in most cultures the serpent is given a very positive interpretation. In India, the cobra, which is a poisonous snake, is a sacred animal. In the Buddhist tradition, the serpent king is next to Buddha in terms of enlightenment. In American Indian cultures, the serpent is revered. The Hopi Indians perform a snake dance taking a snake and placing it into their mouths. This is not an act of courage or of a drug-induced or crazed state of mind, rather it is part of a ritual. This is the way the snake is given a human message. Once the communication is accomplished, the participants let the snake go so it can take the message into the hills. When the snakes return from the hills, they bring the message of nature back to man. In taking the snake into the mouth, the Hopi believe they are able to communicate with nature.

The Bermise have a snake priestess. It's her responsibility to climb a mountain and seek out a den of cobras. When she finds them, she takes one of the cobras and she must kiss it on its nose three times. She does this for the purpose of bringing rain. Because the snake is revered by these people as the giver of life and rain is seen as very intricately involved in the life cycles, the priestess serves a necessary place in the continuation of their existence.

In all cultures and myths, no matter where they come from, no matter when they were penned the serpent is a symbol of continuous life. This is true in the serpent stories of the <u>Bible</u> as well. This may at first be difficult to perceive because for centuries Christian theology has promoted the idea that life is corrupt. Most who endeavor to interpret the <u>Bible</u> find something wrong with life and use the imagery of the serpent as the bringer of sin into the world to support their own ideas. Moving away from theology, let us examine the text as scholars desiring to understand a more productive and positive interpretation of the serpent myth, one in alignment with that found in all other cultures of the world.

Earlier we examined the metaphorical story of Adam, Eve, and the serpent. This is the first reference to the serpent who is actually the primary god in the place called the Garden of Eden. This is probably a new way for you to consider the serpent. In the original text Yahweh, described in most Biblical texts as the Lord God, is described as the spirit of the Lord moving through the Garden. The text does not state that the Garden is Yahweh's home. It is not the Lord's home, he's just a visitor there. It is actually the serpent of the story who knows about the tree of the knowledge of good and evil. It's the serpent who knows what's going to occur in consciousness if the fruit of that tree is eaten. Someone who knows has God-like abilities.

When you study the Old Testament as a scholar, considering interpretations from the original Hebrew, there is nothing indicating that the snake or the serpent is evil. In fact from the original translation, the serpent comes from *Ha-Satan*. Translated into English this means "adversary". To be an adversary does not make you evil nor does it make you wrong. Adversary does paint a picture of being a constant stimulus. Since myths are designed to convey the universality of man's experience and can be personally relevant, we can interpret the snake as a symbol of our own ego, for it is the ego's duty to constantly motivate thinking as we discussed earlier. The adversary is an excellent symbol for this constant motivation. As used in the Old Testament, adversary is a position held by the most beloved of Gods.

Historically, during the time when the Hebrew people moved into the land of Canaan, those native to the area worshipped the Goddess. In mythology throughout the world, the Goddess is often seen in connection with or even paired with the serpent. The serpent symbolizes the mystery of life that comes to fruition through the woman. The Hebrews were a male God-oriented group of people. Their thinking only accepted a male concept of deity. When they moved into the territory of the Canaanites who were worshippers of the Mother Goddess, the Hebrews wanted to exert their authority and control over these people. One of the ways this was accomplished was to banish the belief in the Goddess.

The thinking of the Hebrew is reflected in the way the story of the Garden of Eden was passed down through generations. There is no mention of any kind of the feminine quality of divinity or God. It is only the male aggressive quality that is taught and revered. Yet, as we study metaphysically and we even as we look at our physical life, we know creation occurs where there is duality. It requires both the aggressive and receptive act in order for something to be created. Something to keep in mind when you study the Bible, is to realize that it does come from a specific type of thinking of one culture who shared certain beliefs at a certain time. By combining this information with knowledge from other sources a complete picture can be perceived.

Male orientation dominated the Hebrew society and this is reflected in the stories in the early part of the Old Testament. Because they were intent on excluding this female or receptive quality in the writings, the woman is partnered with the serpent or the snake as being the cause for all the misery in the world.

With investigation we find ignorance of the continuity of life symbolized by the serpent is the cause of misery.

The serpent is also a symbol of creativity. Throughout the Old Testament you hear of serpents and snakes. The second book of the Bible, *Exodus*, tells of the life of Moses. Moses is a man who is ordained by God to lead the Israelites out of captivity in Egypt and into the promised land. His entire life is dedicated to the fulfillment of this pursuit. In metaphysical symbology we recognize this as a parable about the desire to be free of entrapment in the physical. The limitations we create in our consciousness are temporary. There is indeed a different way to think, a different way to live, and a way to expand our awareness.

Moses embodies the very early development in the thinker's ability to use imagination. When he's just beginning to receive the message that he has a purpose to fulfill and a mission in life, there is an interplay between he and the Lord. As the story goes, the Lord appears to Moses in the form of a burning bush. Moses receives the message from the Lord that he needs to go out and rally the people to follow him. This is his mission: to lead these people out of Egypt. Moses is very concerned that the people won't follow him. The Lord responds by asking Moses what is in his hand. Moses has a staff in his hand and he answers, "It's a staff." The Lord says, "Throw it on the ground!" Moses knows when to be obedient, he knows when to heed that inner voice and to follow it so he throws the staff on the ground. Immediately it turns into a serpent. Moses shies away from the snake, and the Lord says "Pick it up by its tail." Because Moses does heed that inner voice, he reaches down and even though he was scared of the serpent before, he lifts the serpent by the tail and it is immediately transformed into the staff. The Lord says, this is going to be your sign for the people. Moses indeed does use this "magic" later. He takes the staff, throws it down, and it turns into a serpent. When he picks it up and it becomes a staff again. The people are amazed and they pay attention to what he has to say.

Symbolically, Moses reveals the knowledge we all possess. The message of his life story is information we gather possess. The message of his life story is information we gather can be transformed through the creation that occurs in our lives. Moses is our ability to expand beyond limitations through the power of imagination. Remember the serpent on one level can be an image denoting creativity.

There's a great legend about a blind prophet named Tiresias. One day Tiresias was walking in a forest and he came upon two copulating serpents. Tiresias took his staff placing it between the two copulating serpents. Immediately he was transformed into a woman. He spent many years as a woman. One day as a woman, he was going through the forest and he came upon two copulating serpents. She took her staff and put it between them and she was transformed into a man. Here we can begin to take another step in understanding the symbology of the serpent. Since the serpent represents creativity, this story conveys the message that whether you are a man (a thinker), or a woman (a conscious thinker), or a man (a subconscious thinker), creativity is the means by which awareness excels, grows, and expands. It requires an act of creation in the conscious mind to gather experiences so we have understandings which transform the subconscious mind. Each time we create, our knowledge of consciousness deepens enriching our awareness of the purpose for existence.

The story about Tiresias continues. There was a time on Mount Olympus when Zeus and his wife Hera were arguing. The issue of disagreement concerned who enjoyed sexual intercourse more, the male or the female? They couldn't really decide because each one only had one-half of the conflict. So they decided to ask Tiresias since he/she was well qualified to answer. Finding Tiresias and asking him the question he replied, "The woman, nine times more than the man." Symbolically, the number nine illustrates completion. A learning experience must be completed for an understanding to be made a part of Self. Understandings aren't gained through postponed or half-hearted efforts in learning. Understandings are gained by full, undivided commitment to learning which causes completion.

The story goes on. When Tiresias said that the woman, nine times more than the man, enjoyed sexual intercourse, Hera struck Tiresias blind. In response to this, Zeus gave Tiresias the gift of prophesy. Symbolically this tells of the opening of consciousness beyond the physical. When we learn to eliminate physical distractions, we birth an opening of perception which we have come to call intuition. It is true that as we use creativity, as we use the serpent, we find ourselves growing in awareness of not only our reasoning capability but also our intuitive abilities. We find that the conscious mind and subconscious mind can work together as a single unit. When their efforts are unified creation occurs.

The serpent is also a symbol of prophetic healing In the Bible this is first described when Moses is having trouble with his followers. Exhausted by their long journey, the followers complain because they lack food and water. The Lord answers their complaints with a plague of seraph serpents who bite the people, killing many of them. This causes the people to turn to Moses admitting their sins and pleading for him to pray to the Lord on their behalf. Moses prays for the people and the Lord responds, *"Make a seraph and mount it on a pole, and if anyone who has been bitten looks at it, he will recover."* Moses makes the bronze serpent and mounts it on a pole. Whenever anyone who had been bitten by a serpent looked at the bronze serpent, he recovered.

How many times have you used your creativity only to find that the fruits of your creativity were less than you expected? Or maybe they weren't anything like what you expected and you considered it a terrible failure or at least a mistake. Because we have this serpent power available to us and we will create either without or with awareness, there are times when we are poisoned by our own use of creativity through ignorance. Ignorance is only a temporary state and it is not part of our innate inner urge, so it only lasts a short time. What at one time was poisoned can be healed. This healing occurs through the use of the serpent power, by creating a new desire that will produce what we want. By transcending our limitations we learn how to use reasoning to discriminate. In this way, we learn to choose our experiences wisely and to choose our creations wisely. We no longer create just for the sake of creating or having, rather we create for the sake of learning to make peace with our Self.

In the New Testament, Jesus rekindles the image of Moses when he says, *"Just as Moses lifted up the serpent in the desert, so must the Son of Man be lifted up. That all who believe may have eternal life in him."* This represents a step in the development of the thinker which happens much later than passages we've investigated. Here man realizes that it's not just in the ability to create that we find awareness, it's not just in the ability to call upon Kundalini energy that we have awareness, rather awareness comes with the recognition that indeed we are thinkers, we are a *Son of Man.* What is most important in any creative endeavor is the evolution of consciousness toward becoming a Christ, *"an anointed, enlightened one".*

Jesus symbolizes the individual who desires to know Self and reach transcendent states of consciousness. As we move from the stories of the Old Testament to those of the New Testament, we find Jesus making many references to Satan and to serpents. One of these is found in Chapter Ten of the book of *Luke.* When we realize that what we are here to do is to use the serpent power, to use creativity for the opening and evolving of our consciousness, something occurs within our own mind. This can be described as a singular purpose. Our vision becomes singular. Our well-being becomes singular. In this story Jesus has appointed and sent out seventy-two representatives to teach truth and inspire spirituality in the masses. When they return they report, *"Master, even the demons are subject to us in your name."* To this Jesus replies, *"I watched Satan fall from the sky like lightning. See what I have done; I have given you power to tread on snakes and scorpions and all the forces of the enemy, and nothing shall ever injure you. Nevertheless, do not rejoice so much in the fact that the devils are subject to you as that your names are inscribed in heaven."*

This story describes the serpent as being a healing power. It is both a responsibility and a privilege to be able to direct that serpent power. Our ability to direct our attention in creation gives us the ability to heal. As long as the attention is singular, we will become whole and complete. The way it describes this here, is *"nothing shall injure you"*. If you are not injured, what are you? You are whole and complete.

Jesus adds, *"Nevertheless, do not rejoice so much in the fact that the devils are subject to you as that your names are inscribed in Heaven."* As we develop a deeper level of understanding and we move our consciousness inward, we come to realize the highest calling of the use of our creative energy is far beyond manifesting a car or a boat or a house or a relationship or a class structure. It's far beyond anything physical. Our driving purpose becomes to manifest light and awareness and to bring out our Christhood, which is illustrated in the stories of Jesus's life. When our vision is singular, we begin to cause our evolution of consciousness to be within our domain. When this occurs the Kundalini truly begins to rise. As the Kundalini rises, we find our healing power is more and more acute, it is more active and it is more accurate. It is demonstrated not only in our perception, but in our directed use of it and miraculous healing occurs. We will discuss this further in the next chapter.

The serpent is also a symbol for the evolution of consciousness. Many of our misconceptions about snakes and serpents and Satan need to be transcended, for this is the only way that you can cure a misconception - transcend the limitations that you have set for yourself. The ultimate word in the English language for that which is transcendent is *God*. God is actually dual in nature. Even though the ancient Hebrews tried to remove any reference to the Goddess in their teachings, it remains there. If you are a Biblical scholar, you know that God said, *"Let us make man in our image."* Us, our, who was he addressing? He was talking to someone. And when that woman eats the fruit from the tree of the knowledge of good and evil, the Lord says, *"we mustn't let man do this or he will be like us. His eyes will be opened, he will be as Gods."* Duality remains in the Old Testament, for those with eyes to see.

God is dual, both aggressive and receptive. In another Hebrew text, the Torah, the word *Malak* is used to conceptualize one part of the duality of God. This signifies his shadow side. Malak is representative of God turned toward humanity. It is a concept that later is translated into the Greek as *Angelos,* meaning messenger which is where we derive the word *angels.* This shadow side of God is the part that communicates with man. The other part of this duality of God is so bright that man cannot bear it. Have you ever heard truth that was just too true to bear? It very painful. Then you've experienced the bright side of God.

This shadow that is representative in the duality in God evolves as you move through the text of the Bible. First it appears as the Word of God. Then it becomes a separate entity almost having free will of its own. It's symbolized as *Lucifer,* who is known as the morning star and the bringer of light. This evolves into Ha-Satan, which we spoke of earlier, a neutral adversary. Then there is a further evolvement into the Satan of the New Testament. Eventually there is the evolvement into the Dragon that appears in the *Book of Revelation.* There is even reference to that morning star once again, and we've gone full circle just like the serpent that eats its tail.

Throughout mythology there is a pictorial image often repeated. This image is of the conflict between the serpent and the eagle. The serpent is bound to earth and the eagle is bound to spiritual flight. Man's destiny is to integrate the two. That integration is symbolized by the dragon or the serpent that has wings. It is beautifully depicted in the *Book of Revelation* in Chapter 12. Here we come to understand in perhaps some of the deepest levels of awareness what this serpent is, why it exists and how it will evolve. The myth begins: *"A great sign appeared in the sky, a woman clothed with the sun and the moon under her feet. And on her head a crown of twelve stars. Because she was with child, she wailed aloud in pain as she labored to give birth.* As we have noted before, the woman represents the conscious mind. She possesses both subconscious and superconscious awareness as symbolized in the moon and sun. Because the conscious mind has gained awareness and control *(crown)* of the inner parts of Self, a new idea is being produced *(the child).*

"Then another sign appeared in the sky." Now both of these are appearing in the sky so these are not just your normal everyday physical type of idea. And it's not your average, normal, everyday kind of conscious awareness either. This is an expanded awareness that includes the superconscious mind. *"Then another sign appeared in the sky. It was a huge dragon, flaming red with seven heads and ten horns, on his heads were seven diadems."* The dragon symbolizes individuality or identity that includes superconsciousness. There is control of the expression of ego in all seven levels of consciousness *(seven heads)* and with the all ten chakras *(ten horns)*. *"His tail swept a third of the stars from the sky and hurled them down to the earth. Then the dragon stood before the woman about to give birth ready to devour her child when it should be born. She gave birth to a son, a boy destined to sheperd all the nations with an iron rod. Her child was caught up to God and to his throne. The woman herself fled into the desert where a special place had been prepared for her by God. There she was taken care of for twelve-hundred and sixty days."* Nine represents the completion of learning experiences. A learning experience is complete when understanding has been attained. This remains universally true no matter where you are on the evolutionary scale of growth. Whether you are a child learning to add a column of numbers or you are attempting to learn how to make your life physically the way you want it to be or you are endeavoring to become enlightened, Christlike, the understanding of how to be a creator must be completed.

"Then war broke out in heaven. Michael and his angels battled against the dragon. Although the dragon and his angels fought back, they were overpowered and lost their place in heaven." In the Hebrew teachings known as the Kaballa there is something called a Seraph. A Seraph is the highest order of Gods angelic servants. The word for Seraphim is the plural for Seraph. The Seraphim are identified with the serpent or the dragon. The name itself is in two parts in Hebrew. *Ser,* meaning "higher being" and *rapha* meaning "healer or doctor or surgeon". Now is everything is coming together? Remember how the Israelites were healed from their serpent bites? They gazed

upon the bronze seraph the Lord instructed Moses to make. The serpent is the symbol of creativity, of the continuity of life, of prophetic healing.

The serpent, Satan, the dragon, Lucifer, each word describes an angel. The Bible describes the angel as having fallen, but still it is an angel nevertheless doing battle with Michael and his angels. Michael is an archangel. His name means who is as God. The word Michael ends in "el" as do most of the archangel's names and the "el" has a similar meaning no matter what language you take it from. In Sumerian "el" means brightness, in Babylonian it means "radiant one", in English it means "shining being". "El" signifies the image of being filled with light, illuminating. This is the goal of mankind, the illumination of consciousness.

Michael is also the viceroy of Heaven. Viceroy of Heaven was actually the title held by Lucifer earlier in the *Bible*. As the stories evolve, Lucifer becomes the Biblical serpent. Therefore Michael and this dragon have similar roots and similar purposes. Chapter 12 of *Revelation* describes the unification of our own consciousness through Michael and the dragon. Here, man transcends good and bad, transcends wrong or right, transcends physical limitations, because his consciousness has been expanded by a singular motivation. *"Then war broke out in Heaven, Michael and his angels battled against the dragon. Although the dragon and his angels fought back they were overpowered and lost their place in Heaven.* Here is the singular illumination, it is no longer dual. *"The huge dragon, the ancient serpent known as the devil or Satan, the seducer of the whole world was driven out. He was hurled down to earth and his minions with him. Then I heard a loud voice in heaven say: Now have salvation and power come, the reign of our God and the authority of his Anointed One. For the accuser of our brothers is cast out, who night and day accused them before our God."* The serpent symbolizes man's ego. We have previously discussed the duty of the ego as a motivator. The ego continues to motivate you toward awareness until you achieve your rightful birthright, until you and I become compatible with the God that brought us into existence. The ego will not stop, because that's its function. The ego does remember the heights from which it has fallen. It remembers that the ideal is illumination, and it will not let you rest until the mind is enlightened. In every level of consciousness, the ego will continue to stimulate you to the heights that are your destiny.

"They defeated him by the blood of the Lamb (always truth) and by the word of their testimony (always truth in action) love for life did not deter them from death. So rejoice, you heavens, and you that dwell therein! But woe to you, earth and sea, for the devil has come down upon you! His fury knows no limits, for he knows his time is short. When the dragon saw that he had been cast down to the earth, he pursued the woman who had given birth to the boy. But the woman was given the wings of a gigantic eagle so that she could fly off to her place in the desert, where, far from the serpent, she could be taken care of for a year and for two and a half years more. The serpent, however, spewed a torrent of water out of his mouth to search out the woman and sweep her away. The earth then came to the woman's rescue by opening its mouth and swallowing the flood which the dragon spewed out of his mouth. Enraged at her escape, the dragon went off to make war on the rest of her offspring, on those who keep God's commandments and give witness to Jesus. He took up his position by the shore of the sea."

Where do we find the expression of the conscious ego? It extends outside the mind, beyond the conscious mind, *"by the shore of the sea"*.

As you endeavor to understand the serpent power, as you endeavor to use her to expand your own consciousness, remember to keep the goal of your enlightenment holy. You can achieve this by upholding the first commandment, by keeping it sacred. The first commandment is "I am the Lord thy God." Keep in mind your reason for existing. This is described in the last chapter of Revelation beginning at verse 12: *"Remember I am coming soon! I bring with me the reward that will be given to each man as his conduct deserves. I am the Alpha and the Omega, the First and the Last, the Beginning and the End!*

Happy are they who wash their robes so as to have free access to the tree of life and enter the city through its gates! Outside are the dogs and sorcerers, the fornicators and murderers, the idol-worshipers and all who love falsehood. "It is I, Jesus, who have sent the angel to give you this testimony about the churches. I am the Root and Offspring of David, the Morning Star shining bright."

There is a wonderful story about the Aztec god of sun and air, Quetzalcoatl. His name means serpent dressed with green feathers. As the legend goes, Quetzalcoatl wore the feather garment to hide his unattractive features. He was the god of wisdom and a teacher of the art of peace. His reign was a period of peace and plenty. His rival, Tezcatlipoce, drove him out by means of his magical powers. But Quetzalcoatl promised to return when needed. He threw himself on a burning funeral pyre and was consumed by the flames. His heart rose to heaven and he was fixed there as the morning star.

May you become the *morning star*. And may you know your own brightness.

The Healing Power of Kundalini

In the Buddhist teachings, the Spiritual aspirant works toward the attainment of Bodhisattva. A Bodhisattva is one who has achieved the realization of immortality yet voluntarily participates in the sorrows of the world. The Bodhisattva knows the principle of compassion underlies the healing principle which makes life possible. Through the development of the healing arts we find a means to remove temporal limitations in thinking which bind consciousness to the physical and blind awareness to our immortality as Spirit. To achieve the state of transcendence Kundalini affords, we must first learn how to dispel these limitations which keep us entrapped and block our soul progression.

Kundalini is known in classical literature as the seat of fire. Described as the serpent, when she is activated the head of the serpent turns upwards, rising through the sushumna and out the crown of the head. As the Goddess rises, she is said to burn her way through any blocks she may find. As we have discussed these blocks can be spiritual, mental, emotional, or physical in composition. Knowing how to identify and release these self-imposed limitations is a prerequisite to consciously activating the Kundalini. A healthy mind and body strengthens expanding consciousness and prepares the Spiritual aspirant for the experience of Kundalini.

Kundalini has enjoyed a relationship with healing throughout man's history. For instance, the symbol of the medical profession is the caduceus. The Latin modification of the Greek *kerykeion* which means herald's staff, the caduceus was originally a magical instrument with two serpents entwined upward around a staff with their heads facing each other. Attributed to Hermes in Greek mythology, the symbol represented fertility, balance, and equilibrium.

Also known as the Staff of Asclepius, the caduceus has endured for centuries because it embodies the essence of health. Named for the ancient god of the art of healing, Asclepius' staff symbolizes man's divinely given ability to produce progressive states of being through the directed use of his creative energy or Kundalini. Because healing is an act of creation, the Kundalini is often referred to as a healing energy, when in reality this is only one way it is useful. For the modern physician, Asclepius' staff is a reminder that the purpose of health is to become whole, to use creativity to replenish life rather than destroy the quality of existing life by only prolonging its duration. For this truth to become a part of man's awareness, every man must respond to his innate ability to create, becoming his own physician by understanding that which lies beyond his physical existence. In this way, physicians must be willing to also become meta-physicians.

I have grown to appreciate choices that souls make when they incarn. This is not something that was always a part of my awareness. When I was growing up, there were times when I felt the pressure of parental authority and believed I would willingly trade my environment for a different one if given the chance. As I matured mentally as well as physically, I opened my mind to knowledge that aided me in building an appreciation for my parents. Probably the greatest knowledge gained was the realization that the choice of my parentage was not the result of some unseen power or chance but rather a result of my own inner desires to excel and grow. My soul chose these two people for the learning experiences they could provide which would accelerate my spiritual progression. This type of expanded awareness changes how you see yourself and how you live your life.

From investigation, I've learned my soul's choice of parents for this lifetime was indeed an educational one. The choice was fortunate in several ways, one of which was a spiritual and supernatural belief in the miracle of healing. My parents taught me that when someone falls ill, you don't automatically call the doctor or run to the pharmacy. Rather, the first thing you do when you are sick is to pray for healing. They taught me the first person you turned to for assistance was not someone physical, it was God. By seeking deliverance from pain through spiritual intervention, I learned to establish a strong connection with the inner power to produce health and wholeness which has served me well throughout my life and made it easier to explore other facets of spirituality.

At the time I was born, my grandfather figure on my mother's side was an evangelist. A hellfire and brimstone preacher, he traveled throughout the country holding tent revivals. Perhaps you have attended such a meeting and your memory including the preconceived ideas it contains is stimulated. Maybe you've seen movies giving Hollywood's perception of revivals and your imagination is conjuring all kinds of images. Some of what you have experienced is accurate, other parts less so.

When my grandfather traveled, he would invite everyone in the town to come and hear God's word as he preached it. He believed in supernatural beings and divine intervention, so I was taught to believe in the supernatural as I was growing up. I was taught to believe in angels and communication from God. I was taught to believe that you could be dedicated to the Lord and fulfill a Spiritual purpose during your life. I was taught that if you lived in accordance with God's laws, the Holy Spirit would guide you in the fulfillment of that purpose. I was instructed that there is life after death, that the physical is not all there is, there is more to come. And I was taught that someone could heal mental and physical afflictions.

Part of my grandfather's revival services included healing with many miraculous results. He was what is commonly
referred to as a faith healer. I witnessed this phenomenon and
was often a recipient of its powerful effectiveness during my
young years. As I grew older I often asked my grandfather how
he was able to heal, because I also wanted to heal and I was
willing to learn how. My grandfather had a hard time giving me
answers that would satisfy my yearning to know. He would
express the source of the power he possessed by referring to the
book he cherished, the Bible.

He would never claim that the power he possessed was
his. He would claim that the power came from the Holy Spirit,
having reached this conclusion directly from the teachings of
the Gospels in the New Testament. My grandfather truly felt
that he was doing the Lord's work in those days, and that one
of those works was to be right with God, as he understood it. He
believed as long as he was true and righteous he could receive
the Holy Spirit into himself and heal the sick. My grandfather
never took upon himself the responsibility that he was the one
performing the healing. He always said that Jesus or the Lord
was doing the healing through him. He was merely an instrument
or channel through which the healing occurred.

In trying to explain this to me, one of the passages he
would cite is found in the book of *Luke,* Chapter 4:14. This
account comes at the beginning of Jesus' ministry when he
returns to his home town. It is one of the first references to Jesus
as a healer, and addresses the source of Jesus's power to heal.
This passage reads: *"Jesus returned in the power of the spirit
to Galilee and his reputation spread throughout the region. He
was teaching in their synagogues and all were loud in his
praise. He came to Nazareth where he had been reared, and
entering the synagogue on the Sabbath as he was in the habit of
doing, he stood up to do the reading. When the Book of the
prophet Isaiah was handed him he unrolled the scroll and found
the passage where it was written: "The spirit of the Lord is upon
me, therefore he has anointed me. He has sent me to bring glad
tidings to the poor, to proclaim liberty to captives, recovery of*

sight to the blind, and release to the prisoners, To announce a year of favor from the Lord.' Rolling up the scroll he gave it back to the assistant and sat down. All in the synagogue had their eyes fixed on him. Then he began by saying to them, "Today this Scripture passage is fulfilled in your hearing." All who were present spoke favorably of him; they marveled at the appealing discourse which came from his lips. They also asked, "Is not this Joseph's son?"

This passage reminds me of my grandfather, because the people who would come to his revivals would be amazed. They would be astounded by his preaching and his healing. They would be surprised and pleased at the results he was capable of producing. They knew that he must have some kind of knowledge that they did not possess, because what he offered was not a common occurrence in their lives. Instantaneous healing was not something they witnessed every day. Yet, in talking with my grandfather he would merely say healing was the result of the Holy Spirit and that you had to be right with God in order to heal.

Being an insistent child, this explanation was not at all satisfying to me. I knew this man, I lived with this man, and I knew him as a man. I knew he was not perfect, and I knew he was a very good man. I also knew from experience that he had this power to heal. Sometimes this power worked and sometimes it didn't, and I wanted to know why.

At first, as an adult searching for the why, I didn't know my investigation into metaphysics would include instruction into mental, spiritual healing. In the practical metaphysics taught through the School of Metaphysics, I was shocked to discover instruction in healing came so early in the course of study. Yet I was excited about the possibility of learning to heal because it was not foreign to my experience. The instruction also answered many of my questions by blending the physical knowledge of how the physical body functions with the spiritual knowledge of why the body operates as it does.

My first teacher of metaphysics was a nurse at a university medical center. Healing was her primary interest, not only in regards to how she had been instructed to physically minister to the sick but also in what she had learned about the mind's power to cause health. Spiritual healing was very important to her, so she would tell us about the class specifically designed for healing before we were even eligible to attend it. By sharing her knowledge and enthusiasm, she fueled my desire to learn and develop in the healing arts.

Another stimulus for my desire occurred shortly after I had begun the course of study in applied metaphysics when my teacher's teacher visited our school. He gave a talk on metaphysics in a room overflowing with people. I was in the kitchen serving as a hostess to our many guests. Between eavesdropping and making sure people's needs were met, I remember leaving the room for a short period of time and coming back to the doorway where the discussion was occurring. The room was absolutely still; you could hear a pin drop. I didn't know what was taking place, so I quickly scanned the room for evidence of what might have transpired to cause such a silence. It was not only a physical silence, but a mental silence. In observing the scene, the teacher was very intently gazing across the room at a young man named Joe. I could tell that not only was the physical gaze intent, but the mental attention was like a ribbon that stretched across the room between the two men. Several times I looked at the teacher and then to Joe trying to discern what was occurring beyond the perception of my physical eyes.

Joe had severe problems with his skin often resulting in boils, and that night he had such a sore on his cheek. As I watched Joe's face, I saw liquid begin to drain, just like a tear, from the reddened and raised sore. When this occurred I knew what was happening, the teacher/healer was using the power of the mind to cause the infection in the body of another person across the room to be released. No one had physically touched Joe. When he had arrived the boil was festering, unopened and quite painful. I was astounded. I hadn't seen the like since the days my grandfather was evangelizing. I had learned some things about the power of the mind, and what I was seeing was in alignment with those teachings. I had enough of a sense of individuality combined with a desire to learn and change, that I knew I could develop the kind of skill I had witnessed with my grandfather and with this teacher/healer.

There was no doubt in my mind. Once I became eligible to attend healing class, I wanted to faithfully pursue the learning and practice available to me each week. The experiences I had with healing class were many times remarkable, yielding results. Sometimes people in the healing class would be healed, and we would see immediate results following the projection of healing energy. Sometimes we would heal people we had never met, and we would receive phone calls or letters from them letting us know how the healing had taken place and what their progress was. Healing was such an exciting ability to learn. It meant illness no longer held a place of authority over man. To know how healing takes place and be able to pass this knowledge on to others, meant freedom from the fear of disease.

Later when I put together what I was learning about healing and what I was learning about the language of mind in understanding dream symbology, I was able to come back to the book I had turned away from for years, the Bible. During adolescence, I had decided I would never understand the Bible and it had come to represent all forms of negativity to me: fear, dread, doubt, sorrow, and guilt. So I didn't even look at the book for years, much less study it. As I expanded my consciousness through disciplined study, I found that attitude was changing. I began opening my closed mind to the truth it had to offer. As I studied the Bible with a keen interest for its universal insights, I began to realize the depth of its instruction concerning consciousness.

By interpreting the Bible in the language of mind, I began to understand how my grandfather had accomplished his healings. In the Gospels, Jesus is described as healing different people with various afflictions. The following story found in the book of *Luke* is called "Cure of the Centurion's Servant".
"When he had finished this discourse in the hearing of the people, he entered Capernaum. A centurion had a servant he

held in high regard, who was at that moment sick to the point of death. When he heard about Jesus he sent some Jewish elders to him, asking him to come and save the life of his servant. Upon approaching Jesus they petitioned him earnestly. "He deserves this favor from you," they said, "because he loves our people, and even built our synagogue for us." Jesus set out with them. When he was only a short distance from the house, the centurion sent friends to tell him: "Sir, do not trouble yourself, for I am not worthy to have you enter my house. That is why I did not presume to come to you myself. Just give the order and my servant will be cured. I too am a man who knows the meaning of an order, having soldiers under my command. I say to one, 'On your way,' and off he goes; to another, 'Come here,' and he comes; to my slave, 'Do this' and he does it." Jesus showed amazement on hearing this, and turned to the crowd which was following him to say, "I tell you, I have never found so much faith among the Israelites." When the deputation returned to the house, they found the servant in perfect health.

When you hear about "faith healing" you need to understand what it is. It is the power that you and I have to create an image in our minds of what we desire. When we use that power to create what we desire, we can expect the manifest likeness of that thought. That's what my grandfather was doing. He, too, thought that he was unworthy so he could not say "I healed". He could only say he was making himself a channel so a greater power than he could heal. That's what happens when you are unworthy. Even in his unworthiness, he had enough faith that this greater power that he could imagine would heal. When he possessed full belief and faith that he was right with his God as he saw it, anytime he wanted to heal, healing took place.

This is the power to create wholeness where dis-ease once existed. As I studied metaphysics, I realized this power has a name and that name is Kundalini. Kundalini is a creative power that all of us possess. References to the Kundalini have yet to enter the mainstream of man's consciousness, so knowledge of her is gained only by those willing to take the time to research esoteric writings particularly those found in Eastern philosophies. Even today, there are very few references to Kundalini in Western writings.

Yet, as I studied I began to realize one of the greatest reservoirs of wisdom concerning man's creative powers is the book I had shunned — the Bible. Among the many universal truths it records, are symbolic descriptions of the Kundalini and man's power to heal. There are two primary secrets involved in our ability to heal. These describe the abilities that man, the thinker, has possessed since he was brought into being. We've always had these, they are not new. These are well described in the language of mind in the second chapter of *Genesis*. Entitled the *"Second Story of Creation"*, this is where our true individuality, referred to in the Bible and other Holy Scriptures as "I Am", is causing creation. This reads in part: *"At the time when the Lord God made the earth and the heavens—while as yet there was no field shrub on earth and no grass of the field had sprouted, for the Lord God had sent no rain upon the earth and there was no man to till the soil, but a stream was welling up out of the earth and was watering all the surface of the ground—the Lord God formed man out of the clay of the ground and blew into his nostrils the breath of life, and so man became a living being."*

The word "man" comes from the Sanskrit word *manu* which is interpreted in English as man. *Manu* also embodies the idea of producing thought and therefore can be seen to signify a thinker. This passage addresses the thinking ability that each individual possesses. In the first chapter of *Genesis* it states that on the sixth day of creation God says, *"Let us make man in our image and after our likeness."* That's the first secret to your ability to heal. The first secret is that you are made *"in the image"* of God, the Creator. This means you are made with thought and by thought. It is thought that makes you alive. To be made *"after the likeness"* means to be like, having similar attributes. Since you are made *"in the likeness"*, you are also capable of creating with thought. If you are going to cause healing where at one time disease existed, you must be able to create an image of health and wholeness.

The second secret of healing is revealed as we read further in *Genesis,* Chapter 2: *"Then the Lord God planted a garden in Eden, in the east, and he placed there the man whom he had formed. Out of the ground the Lord God made various trees grow that were delightful to look at and good for food, with the tree of life in the middle of the garden and the tree of the knowledge of good and bad."* One way of interpreting this passage is to see Eden as referring to the physical existence. For man, the thinker, to use the physical he needs a physical form or vehicle for experiencing. In order for the thinker to cause evolution, he needs centers for creation and their physical counterparts. These are the endocrine glands and brain as symbolized by the trees and the garden. The tree of life would symbolize the pineal gland and the tree of the knowledge of good and bad would represent the pituitary gland.

The passage goes on to explain more about the vehicle that man will be using for his experience in the physical. *"A river rises in Eden to water the garden; beyond there it divides and becomes four branches."* This indicates moving away from the brain out into the body. With the advancement of scientific knowledge over centuries, we know a great deal about the workings of the physical vehicle, or body, man uses. Connections between the brain and the remainder of the body are established through a network of nerves which move from and to the brain. These nerves move through or along side the spinal column in two major systems, the central nervous system and the autonomic nervous system. The *river rising in Eden* is the flow of life force as it enters into the physical body through the medulla oblongata located in the brain stem. This is the point of intake of cosmic energy into the physical body so that it may live. Once the cosmic energy enters your body it becomes life force which is channeled into four systems necessary for physical life.

This passage goes on to describe these four systems. *"The name of the first is Pishon; it is the one that winds through the whole land of Havilah, where there is gold. The gold of that land is excellent; bdellium and lapis lazuli are also there."*

Cosmic energy is made useful to man esoterically through the aggressive and receptive qualities of creation. In this passage, the physical body is symbolized by the *land of Havilah*, Hebrew meaning encompassed and circular. Bdellium and lapis lazuli represent the yin and the yang, the receptive and aggressive qualities. By giving and receiving, pushing and pulling, the cycles of imbalance and balance cause energy to move through what is called acupuncture meridians. Thus *Pishon* symbolizes the flow of energy that nourishes every cell in the body. By study, learning, and practice you can take command of this energy flow releasing any blockages that may exist and establishing the constant flow of life force to every part of your physical body.

"*The name of the second river is the Gihon; it is the one that winds all through the land of Cush.*" *Gihon,* Hebrew meaning formative movement and whirlpool, esoterically represents the part of the chakra system necessary for returning used energy in the physical. In the physical body this energy flow moves through the Autonomic Nervous System. *Cush,* Hebrew meaning firelike, describes the electrical currents flowing through the two neuron chains along the spinal column that innervate smooth muscles, cardiac muscles and exocrine glands. Except to those skilled in esoteric practices, this system remains automatic with most of its functions carried out on an unconscious level of awareness.

"*The name of the third river is the Tigris; it is the one that flows east of Asshur.*" This third expression of cosmic energy esoterically represents the part of the chakra system which recycles used energy back into the inner levels of consciousness. This energy flow is related to the endocrine system in the physical body. The endocrine system works in conjunction with the Autonomic Nervous System to maintain constancy of the body's internal environment. The word *Asshur* is Hebrew meaning level ongoing which aptly describes the action of this energy flow. The Tigris finds expression in the seven ductless glands associated with the major chakras.

"The fourth river is the Euphrates." The *Euphrates,* Hebrew meaning bursting forth and to make fruitful, is the Kundalini energy that you possess. Esoterically, it is the concentrated potential expression of your creative power. In the physical body, this energy flow energizes the Central Nervous System and brain thus enabling the physical to be used by the thinker to promote evolution. Because you have evolved, conscious reasoning is available to you. By responding to your potential, you can exercise your creative power to expand your consciousness and achieve states of enlightenment.

When you learn to use Kundalini energy to enhance your mental creations, you can cause anything that you desire to come into existence. This is why you might be acquainted with the idea of Kundalini energy being used in healing. Healing is produced by dispelling dis-ease and creating wholeness. By replacing nonproductive attitudes with concepts of thinking that are progressive, energies are redirected in the mind and body causing health. The process of changing self-imposed limitations into visionary expansions in consciousness prepares you to receive the benefits of the arousal Kundalini.

From now on whenever you are reading the Bible remember, Euphrates will refer to the Kundalini energy that is available for anyone experiencing Reasoning Man. Later in *Genesis,* the Euphrates is used as a boundary when God gives Abraham the land reaching to the Euphrates. In *Revelation,* you will find the sixth angel pours his bowl on the great river Euphrates which dries up so the kings of the east and the kings of the earth can meet at a place called Armaggedon. You will find the Euphrates mentioned several times in the Bible and now you will have more information concerning what those passages might mean to you.

In understanding healing, it is not until we read the New Testament that the uses for Kundalini energy are described. The point of origin of the thinker is illustrated in the book of *Genesis.* The ensuing books of the Old Testament recount the thinker's journey to what we presently experience as Reasoning Man, a thinker with the capabilities of reasoning using a developed animal-body form. How to use the abilities of Reasoning Man is well documented in the Gospels of the New Testament, so it is there that we discover the steps toward an enlightened use of creation. The life of Jesus and the teachings that lead to the awareness signified by one who is a Christ, teach us how to live as Reasoning Man evolving into Spiritual Man. Healing is presented as a natural step in this evolution.

One of the passages centered on instructions for healing appears in the *Book of Luke,* Chapter 5. In the language of mind, Jesus represents the conscious, physical part of mind that is aggressively expanding his awareness to include the workings of the inner levels of consciousness beyond the physical. In this way, Jesus represents anyone who is willing to cause this expansion of consciousness. Remember this when you read about Jesus. For many people it is easy to believe that Jesus was just a physical man who lived two thousand years ago. Yet the New Testament writings about Jesus' life and actions can also be viewed as an allegory telling us about our own potential.

In the passage called *"A Paralyzed Man Cured"*, more secrets are revealed concerning healing. *"One day Jesus was teaching, and the power of the Lord made him heal."* The individual awareness of the inner urge symbolized by the *Lord* caused the conscious mind to produce wholeness. *"Sitting close by were Pharisees and teachers of the law who had come from every village of Galilee and from Judea and Jerusalem."* You will find as you study the Bible, learning what its symbols mean, that Pharisees are describing people or parts of ourselves that live by the letter of the law. They are aspects that pay lip service, believing one way but acting in conflict to beliefs held, or saying one thing and doing another. You will find that Galilee, Judea, and Jerusalem are more than physical places, they represent places in the inner levels of mind. *"Some men came along carrying a paralytic on a mat. They were trying to bring him in and lay him before Jesus; but they found no way of getting him through because of the crowd, so they went up on the roof. There they let him down with his mat through the tiles into the middle of the crowd before Jesus. Seeing their faith, Jesus said,*

"My friend, your sins are forgiven you." If you are paralyzed, it means you cannot move. You can think that you want to do something or you want to have something, but you cannot cause your physical body to respond in order to have it. The mental attitude that causes paralysis is a stagnation, a refusal to take action and exercise the power of the mind.

I have had the pleasure through years of teaching to instruct many who are working with the zodiacal influence of Scorpio. Most of the people I have met who have a significant Scorpionic placement have placed themselves in some type of limited physical condition. These are usually found in the body such as limited vision or even injuries to the spinal cord. There was a such a young girl I met years ago who at the age of sixteen injured her spinal cord while diving into a pool of water. The cord was bruised causing lack of mobility in her body from the neck down. She started studying metaphysics in one of our Chicago centers, learning about healing and having the advantage of some very good teachers who would not take "no" for an answer. These teachers insisted she become disciplined. Unlike many people who, at a loss for knowledge of something to do that might help, would only offer only sympathy and pity, these teachers made this student move. They would not do something for her that she could do for herself as long as she would try. If she wanted something, she had to put out effort, and even though she rebelled initially, it didn't take her too many months before she was moving from the bottom floor of that school to the top floor. It didn't take her long before she was feeding herself, which she had given up following her accident. It didn't take her long before she was driving, all because she used what she was learning and she had teachers who were using what they had learned. She was learning to cause motion and use the power of her mind.

The key to causing healing is *"my friend, your sins are forgiven"*. We all make mistakes. Metaphysicians don't intend to make mistakes, but sometimes what they do turns out to be a mistake, and they are willing to admit it and make a change. This is when your sins are forgiven, when you are willing to admit the mistakes you have made and make a change so you don't make the same mistakes again.

Sometimes you may have an experience of healing someone only to have them return later with the same disease. This person has yet to have their *"sins forgiven"*. They are still making the same mistakes, producing the same physical disorder. The cause of disease is the error in thinking. When you repent, which means to change, you find you have created health. *The scribes and the Pharisees began a discussion, saying: "Who is this man who utters blasphemies? Who can forgive sins but God alone?"* It sounds like some of my later discussions with my grandfather when I was trying to convince him that he was the one who did the healing and not God. *"Jesus, however, knew their reasoning and answered them by saying: Why do you harbor these thoughts? Which is easier: to say, 'Your sins are forgiven you,' or to say, 'Get up and walk'? In any case, to make it clear to you that the Son of Man has authority on earth to forgive sins"* — he then addressed the paralyzed man: "I say to you, get up! Take your mat with you, and return to your house."*

In the first few weeks of study in the School of Metaphysics, students are taught an exercise called the secret sin. This exercise is a way to admit and identify self-imposed limitations, releasing them from your consciousness so they no longer hold power over you. This is what Jesus is doing here. He is saying admit what you are harboring, because those thoughts you harbor that you are not proud of, that you cannot free yourself from, will cause dis-ease. When you hold onto mistakes without forgiving yourself and making peace, these thoughts will fester in your mind. Allow them to grow in your mind and they will eventually fester in your body as well and you will find you now have disease. The first step in causing a change is to admit those festering thoughts. Examine these realizing whatever they may be they are only evil when you allow them to persist without awareness and understanding. They may be thoughts about something you did when you were six years old! When you were six, you didn't know what you know now. To cause healing you must admit those things you are harboring, those deepest secrets that you think no one else can see. I have found that most of the secrets we believe no one else can see are in most cases the most obvious parts of our expression. It requires a great deal of energy to try to hide them. Don't waste your energy. Become free.

"At once the man stood erect before them. He picked up the mat he had been lying on and went home praising God. At this they were all seized with astonishment. Full of awe, they gave praise to God, saying, "We have seen incredible things today!" Every time you use your mind, every time you use the power of Kundalini to cause healing, incredible things occur. You begin to fulfill prophecy, just as my grandfather believed he was fulfilling prophecy. You begin to fulfill prophecy knowing what the prophecy is *(made in the image)* and why you are fulfilling it *(and after the likeness of God)*.

Jesus addresses one of these prophecies when he speaks to his disciples about healing. In the Gospels, Jesus instructs his disciples differently from how he addresses the masses. The disciples are those who are practicing what is being learned and taught, and in the language of mind they represent the disciplined, controlling aspects of the mind. These are the parts of Self that hold the inner secrets of the power of the mind and its full potential. Members of the healing classes I spoke of earlier are also disciples because they practice discipline of the mind and therefore are capable of offering mental, emotional, and physical healing. The person requesting the projection of healing energy can ask for the type of healing that will benefit his or her individual needs. Some people don't want physical healing, they only want mental healing, so the class projects love and understanding to the individual. With this type of projection the individual has this type of molded thought energy to use to cause peace and contentment in the Self. This is responding to the cause of the person's dis-ease. Just as we can cause healing with thought, we can cause dis-ease from the sins that we hold in our thinking.

There is a passage in *Matthew,* Chapter 13, that describes the essence of what healing is from the point of its origin.   Jesus reveals this through quoting the prophecy of Isaiah.   *"Listen as you will, you shall not understand, look intently as you will, you shall not see. Sluggish indeed is this people's heart. They have scarcely heard with their ears, they have firmly closed their eyes; otherwise they might see with their eyes, and hear with their ears, and understand with their hearts, and turn back to me, and I should heal them."* When you *"turn back to me"*, your awareness is aggressively moving into the inner levels of consciousness.   You are learning who you are and expanding your awareness of who you are becoming. When every activity is caused by a thought of wanting to be close to your God, to become compatible with your God, you cause healing.   The power invested in each of us, the power of Kundalini, is the creative power we use to cause this evolution in ourselves to become a whole, functioning Self and to achieve the state of enlightenment that is our destiny.

With the attention directed toward wholeness, we better prepare ourselves for the transcendental realization of Kundalini, for although you can accelerate healing by learning how to direct her energies through the Brow Chakra keep in mind this is only in preparation for experiencing the fruition of Kundalini. Her final destination lies in the realm of the mystical experience which produces revelation.   Respect her by preparing your Spirit, mind, and body for the enlightenment she will bring.

Courting Kundalini
Preparing the Awakened
Consciousness

The inner urge in Reasoning Man is ever present encouraging progression up the evolutionary scale to Spiritual Man. Each experience beyond the perimeters of the physical plane reinforces awareness of this destiny. Never before in man's evolution has it been so important for man to heed this inner urge and accelerate soul progression. The onset of mystical experience is quickly becoming pronounced and prevalent as more and more individuals rise from sleeping consciousness. As the Kundalini energies make themselves known, the need for Spiritual education for the awakened consciousness becomes essential. Just as the newly reincarned soul needs instruction and guidance for living in a physical body, so the Spirit needs instruction and guidance for productively using the principles of creation.

Thousands of people from all over the world and all walks of life have found the practice of Spiritual disciplines enhance the awareness and use of creative energies. The course of study offered by the School of Metaphysics draws upon these disciplines presenting them to the student in increasingly advanced forms. Although these disciplines are helpful in any creative endeavor, the Spiritual aspirant finds them especially relevant for preparing the mind and body for the onset and use of Kundalini.

We have discussed the prominent uses of creative energy which precede the arousal of Kundalini. Of all of these, the ability to direct the attention in the act of concentration is the most important for it is the cornerstone of any creative activity. The greatest obstacle for creativity is the tendency toward scattering the attention of the conscious mind. When the conscious mind takes no initiative to direct its focus, it is bombarded by physical stimuli and at the mercy of the physical environment. Most of us have learned, many times as a means of survival, how to shut out stimuli. Since this has been accomplished through ignoring rather than choice, we sometimes find ourselves losing track of important details or becoming forgetful.

Many pride themselves on being able to disperse the mind's attention. They claim they can talk on the phone, fill out important documents, and have lunch at the same time. In truth, this does not occur. Since sensory reception occurs in a linear fashion, the brain can only receive and interpret one piece of information at a time. To the practitioner of divided attention it may seem like these events are occurring simultaneously but they are not. They merely exist within the same time period. The conscious mind moves the attention rapidly between what is being heard, seen, felt, tasted, and smelled, accessing incomplete information to and from its computer, the brain.

Later, when the busy executive tries to recall a part of his conversation, he may find himself thinking of soup and salad instead. The memory is garbled. Since he placed the phone call information into the brain with the sensory information concerning lunch, when he wants to draw upon his conversation, the other sensory impressions are remembered as well. He finds he is able to repeat part of the conversation but he also experiences an unknown craving for a tuna fish sandwich.

Rather than strengthening the mind's ability to receive, scattering the attention weakens our ability to respond to situations at hand and later to recall these in detail. Time and money is wasted. Many relationships are destroyed by the mental laziness that causes divided attention. We pretend to listen to others while our attention and therefore our minds are preoccupied with memories or daydreams. When we are "caught" in this state of inattentiveness, we find a hurt or angry partner who decides communicating with us isn't worth the effort since we don't listen.

As a college student unaware of how I was using mind in my everyday endeavors, I would often find my mind becoming distracted while taking a test. Usually, the distraction was part of a song that would repeat over and over, making it difficult for me to keep my mind on the task at hand. Knowing I had a set period of time in which to complete the test only added to my frustration and anxiety. It was not until I began mental discipline exercises in concentration that I realized why this had occurred.

Most of the time I would read and study alone in a quiet room, eliminating as many distractions as possible. However, while living in a dormitory, interruptions were often rampant, from friends dropping in to music sifting through the walls. Sometimes I would stop studying and talk with friends or sing along with a familiar song, but at other times I would endeavor to keep studying while trying to listen to roommates' conversation or while mentally humming the song I was hearing. Since I placed this information in my brain at the same time I was trying to read, later when I needed only the information for the test, I would also remember pieces of conversations or songs.

Although this realization came too late to improve my college study time, it did answer many questions and put to rest any doubt in my ability to direct my mind. It also changed the way I approached life experiences, because it gave me the freedom to use my mind more purposefully. With developed concentration, I found greater control of my attention and will.

Remember, where you were when you heard that President John F. Kennedy had been assassinated? For anyone who was alive and old enough to be conscious of the world around him, that moment is impressed in your brain. You can recall where you were, who you were with, what you were doing; sensory details that usually escape your memory. In the same way, any significant and special event in your life tends to take on the same keeness of recall. These types of experiences occur most often the first time you experience receiving this type of sensory input, and for this reason your mind's full attention to directed to what is occurring thus impressing the full image in your brain. Since the event is fully received and recorded, it is easy to recall details at a later time.

The ability to focus upon a single idea, concept, or physical object frees the mind to fully experience the situation at hand. By choosing to direct thought in a singular fashion, all sensory receptions from an experience can be interpreted and stored as memory for future use. To experience undivided attention is to know something completely from personal experience.

Someone may tell you it is raining outside. You can choose to believe them or not to believe them. Either way, the presence of rain remains a matter of belief for you until you take action that will produce knowing. You might decide to look out a window. Your sense of sight reveals drops of moisture falling from the sky causing wetness on the ground below. When you use your own senses you begin to move from believing to knowing. Using only the sense of sight however leaves you in a state of belief for it will only be when you actually go outside and experience the moisture fully that you will be able to discern if it is rain, mist, or perhaps freezing rain. By using all of your senses, you can make a complete evaluation from personal experience. This is the beginning of knowing. Knowing results in inner authority because you are using your mind to its fullest, taking advantage of the learning your mind affords you.

Concentration is a skill you will use in every area of your physical life. It is necessary in describing any experience thus its practice enhances communication skills. Even more importantly, concentration provides the necessary foundation for effective use of any mental action. From controlling life force in your body to astral projection, from recalling dream communications to living with awareness in the inner levels of consciousness, every mental action requires the developed concentrative skill.

Concentration begins by taking control of your attention. To develop skill in this area, practice fully identifying your experiences. What does the food you eat for breakfast look like? What does it smell like and taste like? What does it feel like in your mouth - hot or cold, smooth or chewy? What does it sound like - crunchy or creamy? Begin to challenge your mind to achieve singular attention, for whatever you place your attention upon is surely worthy of your full attention. What does the music you listen to taste like? It is easy to identify it by sound or feeling. If you read music, it is easy to identify it by sight. But what does it smell like?

As you develop your skill in complete attention, you will find concentration comes easier. Concentration is the willful extension of singular attention. By learning to hold your attention upon a single point for a specific period of time, you move beyond the realm of sensory identification and into the world of contemplation and meaning. Now, the mind is free to think more deeply, enhancing learning. One who is skilled in concentration, will find his creativity quickened. With a concentrated mind, you can choose to develop your ideas without interruption or distraction. This is a necessity for inner talents to blossom.

Practice a concentration exercise daily. To develop your skill, choose a physical object as a recipient of your undivided attention. For a specific time each day, sit relaxed and practice giving your full attention to this object. Should your mind wander, merely return all thought to the object as soon as you recognize you have become distracted.

In the beginning you will find your distractions to be of the physical. Your attention may be drawn to a dog barking, or your arm itching, or someone entering the room. You will find your body and senses will attempt to retain the control you have allowed them to enjoy previously. Do not be discouraged. Keep your ideal of developing a new skill before you. Any time you become distracted, remain relaxed and place your attention where you want it to be.

In time you will begin to separate your consciousness from your physical body and the five senses. You will assert your right to control your body, expecting it to perform as you desire. Physical stimuli will continue around you, but they will no longer hold a distracting power over you. You will remain in control of your attention. This frees you to direct your attention at will where ever you desire. While concentrating, should a need arise in your environment that you want to place your attention upon, you will. This will be from your choice. No longer will it be from the habit of scattered attention.

As you begin to master control of the body, you will begin to gain awareness of another type of distraction. These will be thought distractions. They will interrupt your concentration efforts with memories or imaginings. While focusing your attention, thoughts of what happened earlier in the day or what may occur tomorrow may cause your attention to become divided. When this occurs, note the thought distraction and return the mind sense to the concentration object before you. In time you will learn to still your mind during concentration. When this state is attained, you are ready to begin a spiritual discipline that will elevate your awareness - meditation.

Meditation is both an art and a science. It is the highest expression of communion with creative forces and anyone desiring to raise the Kundalini becomes proficient in its practice. As an art, meditation produces deeper and deeper states of realization. Through daily practice, meditation reveals the continuity of life existing in all of creation. It unifies the consciousness of its practitioner with the vibratory patterns of the universe, freeing his awareness to become whole. It prepares you to meet your maker face to face. And it challenges you to exist in all levels of consciousness, thus accelerating your journey toward compatibility with that maker.

As a science, meditation is a process. Since meditation is the process of going within the mind to inner levels of consciousness, the practice of meditation is always preceded by relaxation of the physical body. Many think relaxation is meditation. Actually, mental and physical relaxation is a process of preparing the mind and body for meditation. Placing the body in a comfortable position with as little muscular tension as possible facilitates the removal of the mind's attention from matters of the physical. Rhythmic breathing also aids by calming the nerves in the body and establishing an even flow of energies. Once the body is stilled, the attention is free to be directed toward its inner work. If you desire to excel in your meditation practice you will seek instruction in the control of your life force.

Meditation requires a focused mind. To meditate, you must be able to focus your attention by choice and at will for meditation is concentration applied toward a single ideal and purpose. In the beginning, direct your attention to the point between the eyebrows, the area of the pituitary gland. Remember your attention is a mental sense and should not be confused with the physical eyes. During meditation, your eyes will be closed thereby cutting off possible sight distractions and your gaze will be elevated slightly above level. Your attention is then placed on your mind's eye.

When successfully practiced, meditation causes an aligning of the conscious, subconscious, and superconscious minds. Regular meditation encourages the expansion of consciousness which precedes arousal of the Kundalini. For meditation time to be productive, conceive a petition or topic for that meditation. Many will relate this to a prayer and having an attitude of Spirituality will aid in deepening your inner communion. Since your ideal is to commune with the Creator and creative forces of the universe, elevate your consciousness toward these objectives when you create your thought form for meditation. By filling your mind with expansive thoughts of love, light, joy, wisdom, and peace you will quicken your ability to still your outer mind and open your consciousness to the inner cosmos. With daily practice, you will find greater rewards with each meditation period. These will come from the expansion of consciousness resulting from the integration of your whole Self.

For progressive meditation, it is best to seek a knowledgeable and experienced teacher. This gives you the advantage of step-by-step instruction of the best way to accelerate your soul progression. A teacher who is skilled in the art and science of meditation will serve as a guide as you move from one stage of meditation to deeper stages. In time, meditation produces the deepened Spiritual awareness which enables the Spiritual aspirant to harmonize, direct, and cooperate with the three principles of mind.

In the beginning, meditation is an inner listening process. Unless you want to listen to the incessant chatter of conscious memories and imaginings, you will want to call upon your developed concentration skill to still your mind. Only by stilling the conscious mind can access be gained to the inner levels of your own consciousness. For this reason, a third practice is also valuable to you - dream work.

One way of stilling the incessant chatter of the conscious mind is sleep. When we sleep, the attention is disconnected from the physical body and five senses. All forms of stimuli can be present around us, yet we remain unaware. A television can be left on, our bed partner might nudge us with an unwelcomed elbow, the room might become uncomfortably warm, the telephone might ring. Any number of events can occur without our conscious knowledge. This state alone does not assist in our desire for Self knowledge because we remain unconscious of what is occurring around us and within us.

While our conscious mind sleeps and our attention is directed inward, two significant events take place. In fact, these are the reason why sleep is necessary. First, sleep enables us to reenergize not only physically, but mentally, emotionally, and spiritually as well. While it is true that our physical bodily processes are slowed during sleep, there is greater rejuevenation taking place within the thinker who uses that resting body. Chakras are allowed to return energy used during the waking hours for the fulfillment of our desires back into the inner levels of consciousness without interference from the conscious mind. As long as the conscious mind is set aside in sleep, it is not creating new desires or reacting to situations habitually thus causing a drag on the energies transformed by the chakras. With the conscious mind aside, the chakras, working under the direction of Universal Law, are free to perform their recycling duty. When we awaken before this process is completed, before the energy has been fully returned, we will experience a tiredness of mind and body upon arising. Even if we have slept a sufficient number of hours to be rejuevenated, we will feel like we "tossed and turned all night".

Attaining proper rest of the mind and body during sleep is another reason to learn how to consciously direct the movement of energies through the chakras. When this ability is lacking in human man, sleep is the only time this recycling can occur unhampered. This process is also the reason why sleep is one of the great curative remedies for dis-ease in human man. Since health and wholeness is the nature of creation, when the limited conscious mind is inactive Universal Laws acting upon the structures of the mind and body will work to correct any illness. This should enhance your understanding and appreciation for rest.

The second significant event during sleep, is the phenomena we call dreaming. Through researching and studying hundreds of thousands of dreams over the last twenty years we, the faculty of the School of Metaphysics, have found two common demoninators in dreaming that universally hold true. One is that every dream is about the dreamer. The second is that every one and every thing in the dream represents specific communication from the inner, subconscious mind to and about the outer, conscious mind. Understanding the universal symbology of dreams is a science that can be learned, studied, and taught. Understanding the significance of the decoded messages is an art that results from practices in developing Self awareness. Every dream will communicate the state of awareness of the dreamer, so investigating the meaning of your dreams accelerates your preparation for Kundalini arousal.

Since childhood, dreams held a special fascination for me. The many questions spawned from my night time dreams are recorded in one of my earlier books. Shortly before I embarked on my journey for Spiritual education and disciplines, my dreams began to take on a different and disconcerting significance. I began having precognitive dreams. These dreams revealed knowledge of events before their manifestation in the physical. For me, prophetic dreaming was another in a long series of diverse experiences resulting from spontaneous arousals of Kundalini. As I progressed in my studies, I realized many times precognitive dreams often occur before, during, or after the awakening of Kundalini.

Begin recording your dreams immediately upon awakening. This will give you a record of the messages from your inner Self. Seek ways to understand the significance of your dreams. Read books on the subject. Take classes. Dreaming is so important it is a major part of the course of study we teach at the School of Metaphysics. The benefits of our study and research are also available through correspondence study. If you have dreams that are precognitive remember they are still about you and endeavor to interpret their inner, spiritual meaning while you investigate their outer significance. Be specifically alert to dreams including theater, plays, television, movies, paintings or artwork, or people involved in these activities. These dream symbols signify creative efforts in your waking consciousness. Should a snake appear in your dream, note its activity and your reaction in the dream towards it. As we have already discussed in previous chapters, the serpent represents use of the creative energies of the Kundalini.

The practice of concentration, the spiritual discipline of meditation, and interpreting your dreams gives you a basis for Self exploration and development. These three provide a means to begin expanding your consciousness and heightening creativity. If you are serious in your desires for spiritual enlightenment you will use these as a springboard for further education in spiritual disciplines. Under the guidance of a spiritual teacher you can excel in your quest for illumination.

The raising of the Kundalini can be the result of spiritual dedication. It cannot be forced but it can be caused through a series of initiations in the expansion of consciousness. Beginning by acquiring concentrative ability, this is followed by learning to direct life force in the physical body. Once the aspirant becomes familiar with these processes he can begin the art and science of meditation which will eventually culminate in the raising of the Kundalini and the experience of transcendent states of consciousness.

The first stage of meditation is stilling the mind and achieving a state of expectant listening. The second stage is characterized by the state of expectant observation and is coupled with the conscious ability to leave the body at will. This is followed by the developed skill of becoming consciously alert during dream states or what is commonly referred to as lucid dreaming. When this is achieved and can be repeated at will, learning to control the life force in the lower chakras is learned and practiced. This is the third stage of meditation. The fourth stage of meditation is inner level travel in the subconscious mind. Utilizing both the conscious and subconscious minds leads to a harmonization of their functions and is demonstrated through the use of intuitive skills such as telepathy and healing. This prepares the consciousness to control the life force in the upper chakras which precedes inner level experience in the superconscious mind. These are the fifth and sixth stages of meditation. From these endeavors the integration of awareness in every level of consciousness can commence. This seventh stage of meditation opens the door to the raising of the Kundalini with understanding. The eighth stage of meditation is the mystical experience we have described. Through repeated mystical experience the aspirant develops mastery learning to function in all levels of consciousness simultaneously which is the final stage of meditation. This is the achievement of enlightenment displayed by all great masters.

It is said that the man Gautama having progressed on his path toward enlightenment encoutered three temptations. The first was the Lord of Lust. This came in the form of three beautiful daughters named Desire, Fulfillment, and Regret. These correspond to our measurement of time as future, present, and past. By releasing attachment to desire Gautama passed the first test and brought to his consciousness the awareness of the ever present now. His second test came from the Lord of Death. Through aligning his consciousness with the infinite Gautama knew his immortality and all the weapons of the Lord of Death turned into flames of worship. He passed this second test by finding the point of stillness within. Upon meeting his third temptation from the Lord of Servitude, the Goddess recognized Gautama's illumined Spirit by addressing him as her beloved Son. In this way, Gautama earned the title of the Buddha for he had achieved enlightenment. By achieving Bodhisattva, Gautama voluntarily participated in the world. It is said he remained on earth as a teacher for the next fifty years.

As each spiritual aspirant reaches toward and achieves the enlightenment of consciousness, he leaves behind the wheel of birth and rebirth graduating from his earthly schoolroom. Karmic obligations are met through bringing understanding of creation to the Self. Through pursuing your destiny as a creator and aiding others in their journey by sharing your wisdom, humanity can evolve more quickly toward our common destiny. In this way the future of the world brightens reflecting the illumined consciousness of mastery.

Transcendence
The Ultimate Power of Kundalini

You are more than you think you are. There are dimensions of your being and a potential for realization and consciousness not included in your concept of Self. Your life is much deeper and broader than you conceive it to be here in the physical. What you are living is but a fractional image of what is really within you. The quest is to know what gives you life, breadth, and depth. This is the essence of Kundalini. When the Kundalini becomes active, the process of revelation has begun.

Your experience is bounded by time and space. Experiences take place in space and in the course of time. Consciously these are determined by the physicalness of man, limiting him to the boundaries of his five senses and the mortality of his own physical body. Subconsciously these are determined by the confines of the soul and the understandings gleaned from lifetimes of physical experiencing. Superconsciously these are determined by the spirit of man beyond temporal experience and crystalized into a state of being and non-being. When full realization is absorbed I Am is experienced. Space becomes a receptacle for timeless creation. We are neither-either, yet both. We have learned to be in the world, but not of it. We have achieved the mystery of being which is everywhere. By revealing the layers of consciousness we come to know the source of our being and cause for our existence as divine and creative beings.

The great quest of man is to evolve as a creative center from which universes and all things come. To exist beyond vibratory creation is to be the Creator of vibration. This is the mystery of the Christian "word" or initial sound. The book of *John* states: *"In the beginning was the Word, the Word was in God's presence, and the Word was God."* The impetus from which the universe was initiated, the big bang is the pouring of transcendent energy into arrangements of space and expansion through the field of time. As soon as this energy enters the field of time, it breaks into pairs of opposites of duality. The one becomes two. With two we discover three ways to relate. One dominates, or the other dominates, or the two are balanced. Thus the two opens the way to the three. Out of these three manners of relationship all things within the four quarters of space are derived and the multiplicity of creation is born. The revelation of consciousness enables the many to become one.

Through reasoning the fundamental structure of the universe can be discovered and consciously experienced. Because reasoning is a sequence of events in the movement of thought, it can be learned and taught. Through intuition this fundamental structure is consciously understood and becomes our being. Because intuition is also a sequence of events in thinking, it can be learned and taught. For the most part this inner sacred knowledge has been in a hands of a few compelled by truth gained in past lifetimes to exhibit the wisdom of the mystic, the charisma of a leader, or the insight of a master. Yet for man to reach his Spiritual destiny, this knowledge must be made available and become a part of the consciousness which so readily accepts the need to teach our children the basics of reading, writing and arithmetic. We must be as willing to teach our youths the Spiritual basics of that which will form the foundation for the expansion of consciousness.

The transcendental state pervades all other states of consciousness. The enlightened consciousness sees the diverse and the unity in everything, never losing the sense of form. No longer is the sensual, material, and temporal world the object of contemplation. The consciousness now perceives something new that has never been known before. The essence of consciousness is revealed. Consciousness becomes reality for the master or mystic whether in waking or dream states. Knowing the secrets of visualization and the qualities of thought which govern energy transformation prepares the thinker to exist and live in all levels of consciousness simultaneously. The integration of awareness in every level of expression of energy produces the transcendent states characterized by Kundalini.

Because spiritual knowledge is more desired than acquired as a state of being, the Kundalini experience begins as a mystical experience produced by a combination of spiritual, mental, and physical factors. Curiosity is awakened in some who hope to gain this awareness by aligning themselves with those who display the brilliance of a more enlightened consciousness. Yet it is not the result of superficial knowledge gained through reading of other's experiences or by associating with someone who demonstrates states of transcendent mastery. At best these serve to fuel the inner desire of the aspirant and feed his curiosity rather than satisfy it. Having discovered the idea of spiritual osmosis lacking in producing desire fulfillment, some move on to seek personal attainment of spiritual states of consciousness only to find that transcendental being is a state of unfoldment and cannot be forced.

The arousal of Kundalini can not be attained through the use of drugs, hypnosis, guided meditation, mantras, or passive sleep states. Although drugs cause a chemically altered state of being in the body and these affect the consciousness, the states they produce are temporary at best and at their worst cause severe side effects not only in the body but in the energies and substance of the mind as well. Some experience such radical chemical and electrical changes that repair can take years if it occurs during a lifetime at all. Hypnosis is the mental equivalent of a drug for the body. It can affect changes in the energies of the mind and can influence subsequent behavior or thought patterns but is temporary in its ability to expand consciousness with understanding. Guided meditation makes the practitioner dependent upon external factors for inner experience thus perpetuating engrossment and identification with the physical. Mantras can focus the mind for a period of time but do not lead to the necessary stilling of the mind required for transcendent states. Passive sleep states, whether dreams are ignored or recalled, leave the consciousness one-sided. With these first efforts for quick Spiritual development, the aspirant finds himself either satisfied through distraction or the desire deepens for Spiritual communion. Whether the desire is satiated or compelled depends largely upon previous Spiritual development in the individual's evolution.

The arousal of the Kundalini is the result of transcendent pursuits through past lifetimes and the present lifetime. It causes an enhanced flow of potent energy to the brain. This produces the possibility of identification of the experience of transcendence. Its effect is easily observed in the creations of the genius and the performance of the prodigy. It is less easily observed in the ecstatic visions of the mystic or the nightmare of those we have labeled insane. Yet each experience is the product of Kundalini in action. By understanding the nature, composition, and function of Kundalini, we can strive to repeat and enhance our effectiveness in its use. We can stimulate and accelerate development of creative genius, we can access spiritually inherent talents and skills for use in our present lives, we can experience states of ecstasy and rapture, and we can identify the unknown calling an end to our nightmarish fears. Through a regular practice of self discipline which leads to self mastery, we can discover the cause and effect relationship of creative mind, prana, and akasha. When development is the result of conscious awareness and will, development can be taught to others. In this way the revelation of consciousness is a process of unfoldment.

Even when sporadic, as it often is in the beginning, the mystical experience propels the awareness into a wider dimension of consciousness which is the destiny of mankind. Kundalini is influenced by conditions both spiritual and material. Environment and personal traits play important roles in the spontaneous experience of Kundalini. The environmental influence of genetic material including so-called smart genes enhances the utilization of the brain thereby increasing its fertility for thinking. Environmental conditions can promote spontaneous arousal of Kundalini through interaction with others. Investment by concerned parents and teachers can offer the skills needed for talent to flourish, but it can just as easily be the desire for escape from outer stimuli which awakens Kundalini.

When the Kundalini becomes active at the time of puberty, she makes herself known in the animal body for physical procreation. The female body experiences the initiation of the menstrual cycle and the male body experience the onset of potent sperm as the result of DNA-coded hormonal changes at the time of puberty. Beyond physical changes, the mind of one open to the arousal of Kundalini may experience spontaneous bursts of energy, uncontrolled and disruptive. These can manifest as uncharacteristic emotional displays, hostility, or depression which cease as quickly as they begin. Often cast off as the throes of adolescence, these spontaneous awakenings go unnoticed, even ignored, and the individual passes into adulthood where the experiences either cease from lack of attention or increase through growing creative urges. There does not seem to be any middle ground.

There is a relationship between Kundalini and physical sexuality. In her resting state, Kundalini is seated at the base of the spine drawing initially on the energies of the Root Chakra. This is why in the first stages of awakening the Kundalini, the sexual appetite may wane. It is also the reason why, for those at the mercy of spontaneous Kundalini activity, sexual activity increases during the times when her illuminating thrust is absent.

During sexual activity the Kundalini energy is drawn outwardly into the act of physical procreation. This stimulates the release of sperm from the male and the release of the ovum from the female for reproduction to occur. Both contain the essence of potential life-giving energies and both are physically mobile through reproductive fluids. Sperm are immediately available at any time for this reproductive function retaining their life-giving essence throughout the lifetime of a male. The evolutionary pattern of the cyclical nature of reproduction in the female enables the physical conditions to be present for procreation. Yet, with the proper mental impetus, an egg can be released and become fertilized at any time, including menstruation. Whether procreation occurs or not, sexual activity provides a means of release for the build-up of Kundalini energy. The demand for generative secretions is so great that there is a need for constant stimulation provided by the erotically pleasing juices accompanying sexual activity.

When the Kundalini is raised the chakra energy is drawn outward, instead of being directed and dispelled into physical activity where it begins to deteriorate, and the energy is channeled up the spinal column. As it rises it draws upon each successive chakra's energy stimulating the vital essence to move up the spine toward the brain. This is the soma referred to in the Vedas, the rosa of the alchemist, the samarasa of the Indian saints, and the Euphrates of the Bible. When energy is being drawn from all chakras it culminates in the mystical experience of Kundalini. This inner balance of duality produces a mystical child, the offspring of transcendent consciousness. The mystical child is often referred to in the Spiritual literature of the world. It appears in the Greek story of Persiphone and the serpent, in the Biblical story of Mary and the virgin birth, and in the birth of Horus, the child the Egyptian Goddess Isis conceived of God. It is said that Buddha was born from his mother's side at the level of the Heart Chakra.

Thus the divine urge which brings a child into being drives that child at a certain period in his life toward the act of procreation. When the time is ripe, he is filled with the urge for Self awareness as he was once filled with erotic desire. This is why the final phase of the four stages of man is characterized by wisdom.

Personal traits play an equal if not more important role in the spontaneous activation of Kundalini for they constitute the Spiritual composition of the individual. These traits are dual in nature. Some are the result of understandings gained in previous lifetime experiences. These are the talents we have from birth constituting the areas of giftedness or genius. The wealth of experience in creativity continues through our spiritual experience spanning the thousands of physical years in the earth plane. They press from within, seeking expression and paving the way for the experience of Kundalini. Finding a fertile consciousness they will grow and express becoming a propelling force for Kundalini as they mingle with what is learned in the present lifetime. Thus for those viewed as creative geniuses the experience of Kundalini was imminent.

Personal traits that are developed in the present lifetime also cultivate consciousness for the manifestation of Kundalini. Many of these we have discussed as spiritual practices and disciplines in previous chapters. Whenever healthy attitudes and actions are nurtured, consciousness experiences the freedom to create and expand. The repeated experience of quiet meditation time taught by many religions produces an acquaintance with the stilled mind which prepares the way for Kundalini arousal. Early discipline in the cultivation of a skillful talent such as playing a musical instrument, or singing, or dancing, or athletics, develops the concentration and creativity. Fostering self betterment develops traits of steadfastness and excellence characteristic of spontaneous arousals of Kundalini. Love and encouragement feed the inner desire to learn and grow, yielding a harvest of creative activity leading to the realization of oneness experienced in transcendent states.

When knowledgeable guidance is missing, the mystical experiences produced by the aroused Kundalini are transient giving rise to disorientation and confusion due to a lack of understanding. The brilliant artist experiences inspiration bursting from some unknown source only to experience its immediate cessation. The artist is left feeling empty and helpless to direct these fleeting flirtations with expanded consciousness. At a loss to identify and understand his own thinking processes, he attributes these bursts of inspiration to an unknown source. Ill equipped to respond to the demands of spontaneous arousal, the world is filled with Poes, Doyles, Fitzgeralds, and Hemingways all creative geniuses who experienced deep depressions following spurts of visionary endeavors and who sought escape in drugs or alcohol rather than pursue the meaning and control of their own expansive creativity.

Others experiencing Kundalini attribute it to some unseen supernatural and unknown power. The devoutly religious, having lived in thought and deed according to the moral dictates they believe in, experience the same kind of confusion when some unforeseen occurrence such as the seemingly meaningless death of an innocent child leads them to expand their mind to question the motives of a benevolent God. Many banish spirituality from their lives, disavowing any connection with a greater power or order in the universe becoming engrossed in the limitations of the physical rather than moving beyond self-imposed limitations in their concepts of the divine.

Through understanding the duality of our existence and integrating the facets of our consciousness man can expect to discover answers to the mysteries of his universal experience. The answers were not found in the limitations of the past and trying to return to living in that past produces stagnation. Only by moving forward in knowledge and experience can we move beyond spontaneous arousal of Kundalini and toward the enlightenment of transcendent consciousness. For the enlightened, the universe of spirit and the world of forms coexist without confusion and the Kundalini becomes a spiritual creative force for the acceleration of mankind.

Pursuit of transcendence through the use of Kundalini prepares the way for the evolution of animal man into spiritual man. This begins when temporal goals are replaced with spiritual goals. For 200 years, science has excelled in expending the earth's resources. Had the discipline of Kundalini been made earlier, the state of the world and experience of humanity would now be vastly different. When the Kundalini is active in aware individuals there will be planning with intuitive foresight, wholistic and healthy conditions, unity in mankind's thought which will stimulate advancement in social and political order. This can only be achieved through widespread awareness of the destiny of man as a thinking being and of the purpose for physical existence combined with the means to achieve it.

There are two products of an active Kundalini: those men and women who are enlightened having achieved the state of illumination and those who possess and demonstrate genius and talent. These comprise the two main classes of human beings responsible for every advance made by mankind thus far. As the nature of Kundalini and the importance of the transcendental consciousness becomes common knowledge, its acceptance can cause a revolution in current scientific research and endeavors. The universe is a creation of consciousness. What we perceive with the five senses is merely one dimension of many. The leaders of our time are advanced in quick thinking in their realms of endeavor far surpassing the greatest thinkers of our past. Yet many of these are severely deficient and handicapped when compared to the spiritual masters of our past for they seek the fulfillment of temporal goals only. Only when this quick thinking can be balanced with awareness of the Spirit will there be a means to offset an overinflated ego and the boundless greed of the highly intelligent mind. We must come to realize that the beckoning of Kundalini is an invitation for the revelation of our consciousness and the acceleration of spiritual development. Only by accepting our ability to respond to her may we hope to achieve true humanitarian progress.

The Mystical Experience and Ecstasy

The means to accomplish the wholistic development of man is contained in the spiritual literature of the world and demands the advancement of scientific investigation. Whatever petty egotism may arise in the minds of scientific or religious adherents must be transcended so the full scope of man's potential may be identified and realized through the joining of their efforts for the betterment and acceleration of mankind. The religious must transcend the limitations of the unseen and the scientist must transcend the limitations of what is seen. The mystical experience must be viewed by both as a point of origin for further spiritual and physical investigation.

To see the mystical experience as purely of a religious nature is at best a mistake in judgement. Mystical experiences arise from creative impulses in the mind and are the results of a consciousness which is growing. Every genius gifted with creativity stands at the threshold of universal consciousness. Once he or she crosses into this new dimension, his or her vision and experience come together. Mystical experiences are characterized by this unifying of individual consciousness with the cosmic consciousness.

Mystical experiences associated with the spontaneous and unconscious raising of Kundalini are accompanied by an altered sense of time and space. The experience itself is usually short in physical time duration but can seem to last for much longer because it is a state of being. The most pronounced part of the experience is the sensation of light emanating through and around the consciousness. It is as if the mind and indeed the brain are illumined and everything perceived is luminous. Often harmonious configurations of sound are experienced including the vibratory hum, or from esoteric Hindu teachings the Om, of creation. These are accompanied by extraordinary insights and new depths of knowledge as the aspirant experiences glimpses of other planes of existence. The visions impressed in the consciousness result in a spiritual exaltation vaguely reminiscent of sexual orgasm.

When first experienced, Kundalini can be spontaneously active appearing to come and go by some unknown will. One who cultivates his desire to know and understand his experiences undergoes a progression of development with each successive experience with Kundalini. Earlier Kundalini experiences bring a fluency in expression, vast knowledge and deep insights to Spiritual aspirants. They have access to understandings and flashes of insight uncommon to the average man. They tend toward a wholistic construction of ideas blending spiritual principles with physical factors, as a result many of their ideas are innovative for society. The benefits of their expansion of consciousness is shared with many, for spontaneous awakenings of Kundalini propel the individual toward greater and greater acts of creation far beyond the confines of his own limited space. Welling from within, the energy must be expressed, understood, and shared in a manner befitting its qualities of revelation. If the individual fails in this, the Kundalini will again sleep and another lifetime will pass.

When one responds to the awakening of Kundalini, he or she finds repetitions of the mystical experience occurring throughout the life. As the experience of Kundalini recurs, the individual becomes more determined and reliable. His thinking becomes directed and increasingly insightful so he is well respected and often sought out for counsel. He holds and lives by a high regard for truth, altruism, and self mastery. These qualities aid the individual to adjust to the changes an awakened Kundalini demands.

As the Kundalini becomes more active, the individual may experience changes in thinking and behavior. As consciousness expands he will respond according to the greater awareness. What was previously important to him may no longer arrest his attention. For instance, the desire for newness which at one time manifested in desires for a new car, a new relationship, or a new position of authority now finds its expression in a desire for new thoughts, new insights, and new revelations. Someone who at one time had to be surrounded by people for stimulation may now experience a preference for solitude and quiet. One who had a me-first attitude now finds a diminishing of the insecure ego and the blossoming of a Self centered generosity.

The impulse toward Self introspection strengthens as one adjusts to the experience of Kundalini. This is coupled with a repeated urge to meditate or pray as a means to establish and deepen connections with inner resources and the inner source. This in turn produces a sustaining inner peace which replaces attachment to the temporal and sensory world. By enhancing contact with the spirit, a greater regard for principles and universality is integrated into the consciousness. This produces a growing love and compassion for all of mankind which wells up from within the Spiritual aspirant.

Throughout the world man has described the mystic experience. Whether in Siberia or the Americas, shamans live and teach of spiritual unfoldment. A shaman can be male or female. Late in childhood or during the early youth, near the onset of puberty and activation of the Kundalini, each has an overwhelming experience which turns him totally inward. What was unconscious becomes conscious. It is a mystic experience which begins the shaman on his path. The shaman's power is significant because unlike a special order of priests devoted to a deity, the shaman's power symbolized his own personal experience of deity. This personal experience of deity is part of the universal mystic experience of Kundalini.

Mystic experience is sometimes the result of cultural ritual. A Bushman society living in the desert practices a trance dance. There life is physically challenging and they live with males and females separated. They only come together in the dance. The women form a circle, beating their thighs to set a rhythm for the men who dance around them. The women control the dance through their singing because they are viewed as representative of life. Men are seen as the servant of life. The men circle, dancing well into the night, until one man passes out. He experiences a flash similar to a lightning bolt passing from his pelvic area up the spine into the head.

The mystical experience of Kundalini has traditionally been described as ecstasy. When the pairs of opposites are transcended man surpasses his dual nature becoming one. In effect he dies to the flesh and is born into Spirit. His identity becomes consciousness and life and he is keenly aware of the one radiance shining through all of creation. The bliss accompanying this ecstasy is nature's incentive for the effort directed toward Self transcendence, just as orgasm is the incentive for reproduction.

Spiritual rebirth is the essence of ecstasy. It is the direct experience of inspiration and revelation, of light and sound, and of bliss or inner happiness. In Hindu teachings there are three Sanskrit words reflecting the mystical experience of ecstasy. *Sat* represents being, *Chit* embodies consciousness, and *Ananda* meaning bliss or rapture. These three exemplify the transcendent consciousness attained in mystical experience.

Mystical experience can be and is described in the Spiritual literature of the world. There are several qualities which comprise the state of ecstasy reached when the Kundalini is raised. The most impressive of these is a vivid sensation of light. During the experience the whole being becomes illumined and every part of creation seems to shimmer. The Bhagavad Gita describes it in this way: *"Those who employ their minds constantly in contemplation of the Real Self and thus are restrained from superfluous desires find freedom from the attraction of the pairs of opposites. They are delivered from pleasure and pain and are thus relieved of confusion and illusion. They ascend to that plane which endures forever. They pass on to a place which is not lighted by either the sun or the moon, not even by fire, but which is radiant beyond imagination."* The radiance spoken of is the emanation of the illumined consciousness. During the experience, the mystic or Spiritual aspirant even assumes a radiant appearance which can last far beyond the mystical experience itself.

The second quality of the mystic experience is harmonious sound. This is the reception of the vibration of the universe. It is direct knowledge of the movement of creation. The *Chandogya Upanishad* states: *"The essence of all beings is earth, The essence of earth is water, The essence of water is plants, The essence of plants is humanity, The essence of humanity is speech, The essence of speech is sacred poetry, The essence of sacred poetry is music, The essence of music is Om, The best of all essence, the highest, Deserving the highest plea, the Eighth."* The mystical experience unites the consciousness of Self with the consciousness of the cosmos. This can only be known by releasing the separateness of self consciousness by entering into the transcendence of the cosmic consciousness.

Third is a feeling of consummate rapture and joy. John writes in the book of *Revelation*: *"On the Lord's day I was caught up in ecstasy."* Transcendence produces this profound sense of rapture which can most easily be described as thrill. Reminiscent of falling in love, the mystical experience embodies the love which courses throughout the universe in the fiber of all creation. The *Dhammapada* states: *"Health, contentment and trust are your greatest possessions, and freedom your greatest joy. Look within. Be still. Free from fear and attachment, know the sweet joy of the way. How joyful to look upon the awakened and to keep company with the wise. How long the road to the man who travels with a fool. But whoever follows those who follow the way discovers his family, and is filled with joy. Follow then the shining ones, the wise, the awakened, the loving, for they know how to work and forbear."* The joy experienced in the transcendent state wells from within having no beginning or end. It is the innate and unpremeditated response to the boundless love of your maker as it flows through universal consciousness.

This produces the fourth quality of the mystical experience. There is an overwhelming sense of intimacy with an infinite presence or celestial being. The old consciousness which perpetuated barriers is released opening the consciousness to the new resurrected awareness of eternal life. The book of *Luke* gives an account of the final moments of the life as Jesus: *"The curtain of the sanctuary was torn in two. Jesus uttered in a loud cry and said, 'Father, into your hands I commend my spirit'."* Following the mystical experience there is a constant inner awareness of a connection with that which is omnipresent and omniscient. A constant and inner urge toward the divine pervades consciousness.

Fifth is a sense of the union with an infinite source of all knowledge. By unifying consciousness with the essence of creation, the point of origin is revealed. The Tao Te Ching describes this: *"All things arise from Tao. They are nourished by Virtue. They are formed from matter and shaped by environment. Thus the ten thousand things all respect Tao and honor Virtue. Respect of Tao and honor of Virtue are not demanded, but they are in the nature of things. Therefore all things arise from Tao and by Virtue they are nourished, developed, cared for, sheltered, comforted, grown, and protected. Creating without claiming, doing without taking credit, guiding without interfering, This is Primal Virtue"*. When immersed in cosmic consciousness the Spirit awakens to the dynamic power which feeds the universe. The source of all being is known.

An innocent sense of wonder and awe at the vision received is the sixth quality of the mystical experience. Again, the Tao states: *"In caring for others and serving heaven, there is nothing like using restraint. Restraint begins with giving up one's own ideas. This depends on Virtue gathered in the past. If there is a good store of Virtue, then nothing is impossible. If nothing is impossible, then there are no limits. If a man knows no limits, then he is fit to be a ruler. The mother principle of ruling holds good for a long time. This is called having deep roots and a firm foundation. The Tao of long life and eternal vision."* A profound sense of worthiness arises from within and fills the being. The vision of the mystical experience transcends those of earlier inner level experiences which preceded the arousal of Kundalini. This vision is unfolding of the illumined consciousness.

Seventh is tears at the sublime sense of being. One of several reactions in the body to the mystical experience, crying is a manifestation of these changes in consciousness. Mohammed wrote in the Koran: *"When the sun ceases to shine; when the stars fall down and the mountains are blown away; when camels big with young are left untended and the wild beasts are brought together; when the seas are set alight and men's souls are reunited; when the infant girl, buried alive, is asked for what crime she was slain; when the records of men's deeds are laid open and the heaven is stripped bare; when Hell burns fiercely and Paradise is brought near; then each soul shall know what it has done."* Uniting with cosmic consciousness causes immediate alterations in the substance of the Spirit, mind, and body.

The illumination of perpetual wisdom shines from without and within and is the eighth quality. It is said the Norse god Odin had two wolves crouched at his feet and two ravens perched on his shoulders. Each day the ravens would fly though the world and bring back reports of what men would do. The name of one raven was thought and the other was named memory. While the other gods feasted, Odin pondered what thought and memory taught him. Odin was the All Father, the supreme among gods and men yet he constantly sought wisdom. He journeyed to the Well of Wisdom hoping to discover that which eluded him. Reaching the Well he found it guarded by Mimin the wise and he begged for a draught from the Well. When Mimin answered he must pay for it with one of his eyes, he consented to lose the eye in order to gain wisdom. Transcendence is known by those with singular perception, and by those the wisdom of the universe is perceived.

When the Lord told Solomon he would give him whatever he requested, Solomon asked for an understanding heart to judge the Lord's people and to know right from wrong. To this the Lord replied, *"Because you have asked for this - not for a long life for yourself, nor riches, nor for he life of your enemies, but for understanding so that you may know what is right - I do as you requested. I give you a heart so wise and understanding that there has never been anyone like you up to now, and after you there will come no one to equal you."* The transcendental experience produces the wisdom of Solomon and the fulfillment of all desires which leads to enlightenment.

The ninth and final quality of the mystical experience is the revelation of the divine in creation. The Dhammapada states: *"Better than a hundred years of mischief is one day spent in contemplation. Better than a hundred years of ignorance is one day spent in reflection. Better than a hundred years of idleness is one day spent in determination. Better to live one day wondering how all things arise and pass away. Better to live one hour seeing the one life beyond the way. Better to live one moment in the moment of the way beyond the way."*

The early mystical experiences of Kundalini begin the illumination that will culminate in mastery. All great Spiritual masters have described this state. Jesus, Gautama, Zarathustra, Shankaracharya, Mohammed and others throughout history have experienced pure consciousness and entered enlightenment. By receiving instruction and mastering the Self, each learned the secrets of Kundalini by being awake in consciousness at all times. This is the destiny of all mankind.

The momentary experience of ecstasy beckons man to transcend his physical, temporal and animal existence and enter into the realms of cosmic consciousness to face his immortality. Endeavor to rouse your sleeping consciousness developing respect for your creative abilities and cultivating their wise use. Heal your Self of limitations in thinking and bodily restrictions. Invest your time and energy into pursuits that will feed your soul and accelerate your evolutionary development. Be faithful in any spiritual discipline. Be alert to indications of the mystical experience of an aroused Kundalini. Strive to develop your mind and Spirit so you are prepared when she beckons you. When she enters your consciousness, court her. Give her your love, and time, and attention. She will repay your kindness a thousandfold.

About the Author

A teacher, wife, mother, futurist, counselor, minister, intuitive reporter, editor, artist, composer, singer, designer, poet, administrator, media consultant and producer, Barbara Condron lives what she teaches. She, her husband Daniel, and others committed to teaching the fine art and science of Multidimensional Consciousness, are actively envisioning and manifesting a College for Intuitive, Spiritual Man. They currently live on the campus in Southwestern Missouri with their son Hezekiah and an ever-evolving group of students from around the world.

Additional titles available from SOM Publishing include:

Every Dream is about the Dreamer by Dr. Barbara Condron
  ISBN: 0944386-27-X $13.00
Peacemaking: 9 Lessons for Changing Yourself, Relationships, & World
  Dr. Barbara Condron   ISBN: 0944386-31-8 $12.00
The Tao Te Ching Interpreted & Explained
  Dr. Daniel R. Condron ISBN: 0944385-30-x $15.00
How to Raise an Indigo Child
  Dr. Barbara Condron   ISBN: 0944386-29-6 $14.00
Atlantis: The History of the World Vol. 1
  Drs. Daniel & Barbara Condron ISBN: 0944386-28-8 $15.00
Karmic Healing by Dr. Laurel Clark ISBN: 0944386-26-1 $15.00
The Bible Interpreted in Dream Symbols - Drs. Condron, Condron,
  Matthes, Rothermel   ISBN: 0944386-23-7 $18.00
Spiritual Renaissance– Elevating Your Conciousness for the Common Good
  Dr. Barbara Condron   ISBN: 0944386-22-9 $15.00
Superconscious Meditation - Kundalini & Understanding the Whole Mind
  Dr. Daniel R. Condron   ISBN 0944386-21-0 $13.00
First Opinion: Wholistic Health Care in the 21st Century
  Dr. Barbara Condron   ISBN 0944386-18-0 $15.00
The Dreamer's Dictionary
  Dr. Barbara Condron ISBN 0944386-16-4 $15.00
The Work of the Soul
  Dr. Barbara Condron, ed. ISBN 0944386-17-2 $13.00
Uncommon Knowledge: Past Life & Health Readings
  Dr. Barbara Condron, ed. ISBN 0944386-19-9 $13.00
The Universal Language of Mind – The Book of Matthew Interpreted
  Dr. Daniel R. Condron   ISBN 0944386-15-6 $13.00
Permanent Healing
  Dr. Daniel R. Condron   ISBN 0944386-12-1 $13.00
Dreams of the Soul - The Yogi Sutras of Patanjali
  Dr. Daniel R. Condron   ISBN 0944386-11-3 $9.95

To order write:
  School of Metaphysics
  World Headquarters
  163 Moon Valley Road
  Windyville, Missouri 65783   U.S.A.

Enclose a check or money order payable in U.S. funds to SOM with any order.
Please include $4.00 for postage and handling of books, $8 for international
orders. A complete catalogue of all book titles, audio lectures and courses, and
videos is available upon request.
Visit us on the Internet at *http://www.som.org*   e-mail: som@som.org

About the School of Metaphysics

We invite you to become a special part of our efforts to aid in enhancing and quickening the process of spiritual growth and mental evolution of the people of the world. The School of Metaphysics, a not-for-profit educational and service organization, has been in existence for three decades. During that time, we have taught tens of thousands directly through our course of study in applied metaphysics. We have elevated the awareness of millions through the many services we offer. If you would like to pursue the study of mind and the transformation of Self to a higher level of being and consciousness, you are invited to write to us at the School of Metaphysics World Headquarters in Windyville, Missouri 65783.

The heart of the School of Metaphysics is a four-tiered course of study in mastering consciousness. Lessons introduce you to the Universal Laws and Truths which guide spiritual and physical evolution. Consciousness is explored and developed through mental and spiritual disciplines which enhance your physical life and enrich your soul progression. For every concept there is a means to employ it through developing your own potential. Level One includes concentration, visualization (focused imagery), meditation, and control of life force and creative energies, all foundations for exploring the multidimensional Self.

Experts in the Universal Language of Mind, we teach how to remember and understand the inner communication received through dreams. We are the sponsors of the National Dream Hotline®, an annual educational service offered the last weekend in April. Study centers are located throughout the Midwestern United States. If there is not a center near you, you can receive the first series of lessons through correspondence with a teacher at our headquarters.

For those desiring spiritual renewal, weekends at our Moon Valley Ranch offer calmness and clarity. Spiritual Focus Weekends center around a theme – kundalini, genius, meditation, influence – or explore marriage, parenting, or your purpose in life. Each includes an intuitive report designed for the session and given in your presence. Mentored by College instructors and Psi counselors, these weekends are experiences in multidimensional awareness.

The Universal Hour of Peace was initiated by the School of Metaphysics at noon Universal Time (GMT) on October 24, 1995 in conjunction with the 50th anniversary of the United Nations. We believe that peace on earth is an idea whose time has come. To realize this dream, we invite you to join with others throughout the world by dedicating your thoughts and actions to peace through reading the *Universal Peace Covenant* as ONE VOICE at midnight December 31st. Living peaceably begins by thinking peacefully. Please contact us about how you can participate.

There is the opportunity to aid in the growth and fulfillment of our work. Donations supporting the expansion of the School of Metaphysics' efforts are a valuable way for you to aid humanity. As a not-for-profit publishing house, SOM Publishing is dedicated to the continuing publication of research findings that promote peace, understanding and good will for all of Mankind. It is dependent upon the kindness and generosity of sponsors to do so. Authors donate their work and receive no royalties. We have many excellent manuscripts awaiting a benefactor.

One hundred percent of the donations made to the School of Metaphysics are used to expand our services. Donations are being received for Project Octagon, the first educational building on the College of Metaphysics campus. The campus is located in the beautiful Ozark Mountains of Missouri. This proposed multipurpose structure will include an auditorium, classrooms, library and study areas, a cafeteria, and potential living quarters for up to 100 people. We expect to finance this structure through corporate grants and personal endowments. Donations to the School of Metaphysics are tax-exempt under 501(c)(3) of the Internal Revenue Code. We appreciate any contribution you are free to make. With the help of people like you, our dream of a place where anyone desiring Self awareness can receive wholistic education will become a reality.

We send you our Circle of Love.

Please call or write for your copy of the
UNIVERSAL PEACE COVENANT

or visit
www.peacedome.org